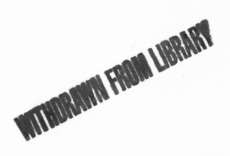

APPLIED MEDICAL GEOGRAPHY

SCRIPTA SERIES IN GEOGRAPHY

Series Editors

Richard E. Lonsdale ● Antony R. Orme ● Theodore Shabad

Shabad and Mote · Gateway to Siberian Resources, 1977

Lonsdale and Seyler · Nonmetropolitan Industrialization, 1979

Rodgers · Economic Development in Retrospect, 1979

Dienes and Shabad · The Soviet Energy System, 1979

Pyle · Applied Medical Geography, 1979

APPLIED MEDICAL GEOGRAPHY

Gerald F. Pyle
The University of Akron

1979

V. H. WINSTON & SONS
Washington, D.C.

A HALSTED PRESS BOOK

JOHN WILEY & SONS

New York   Toronto   London   Sydney

V. H. Winston & Sons, a Division of Scripta Technica, Inc., Publishers
1511 K Street, N.W., Washington, D.C. 20005

Distributed solely by Halsted Press, a Division of John Wiley & Sons, Inc.

Library of Congress Cataloging in Publication Data:

Pyle, Gerald F.
    Applied medical geography.

    (Scripta series in geography)
    1. Medical geography.   I. Title.   II. Series:
[DNLM: 1. Epidemiology.   2. Geography.   WB700
P996a]
RA792.P94   1979   614.4'2   78-27856
ISBN 0-470-26643-0

Composition by Isabelle Sneeringer, Scripta Technica, Inc.

To the memory of
Lettie Lindley Wood

CONTENTS

PREFACE

I should like to extend my warm thanks to the many generous people who helped make this book possible.

Victor Winston's willingness to incorporate a volume considered a "rare event" by many geographers in the Scripta Series in Geography is greatly appreciated. I should also like to thank Victor for his understanding of the time-consuming efforts entailed in developing a text on medical geography. In retrospect, writing a book about medical geography can be more exhausting than "exhaustive." As a result, I drew upon my own experiences and strengths in medical geography research, no doubt at the expense of some concepts necessary to understanding the geography of human health problems. The latter approaches include illness behavior, cultural determinants of health problems and malnutrition. Gary Shannon's forthcoming works on the geography of illness behavior should be of supportive assistance to the reader of this book, and I suspect Melinda Meade's future contributions in the area of disease and culture can assist in filling that void. In addition, Andrew Learmonth's recent exposition of the geography of disease and hunger places malnutrition into an important spatial context.

Most of this book was written in conjunction with my academic appointment at The University of Akron. Its completion would not have been possible without the generous and hospitable support of Claibourne Griffin, Dean of the Buchtel College of Arts and Sciences. Likewise, important administrative and intellectual support were tendered by Edward Hanten and William Hendon, of Urban Studies. Judith Sherman demonstrated her continued unswerving loyalty through the typing of various drafts and the completed manuscript. My thanks go to Joan Gossner for her dedicated efforts as a graduate research assistant performing many supportive tasks. Vicky Hosler and Robert Cook deserve credit for coordinating much of the data processing involved in the development of this work. The maps and other illustrations were developed under the supervision of Duane Neimeyer with the assistance of William Butler. The glossary of health planning terms was adapted from information supplied by the Health Planning and Development Council of Wooster, Ohio due to the kind assistance of Mr. Robert Linstrom.

Some of the early phases of research and writing contained within this work were accomplished while I was a visiting academic at the University of South Carolina. I am indebted to Julian Minghi and David Cowen for their un-questioning support in making important resources of the Department of Geography available. My appreciation is also extended to several who were graduate students in geography at that time, including Lynn Shirley and Ann McGirt. Cooperation from the School of Public Health at the University of South Carolina included constructive criticisms offered by Robert Lewis and data analysis assistance accomplished by Barbara Hegler. One reason for the inclusion of examples of health conditions in various parts of South Carolina is the exceptionally warm reception given to techniques in spatial analysis by my friends at the South Carolina Department of Health and Environmental Control. It was Michael Loving's idea that I examine the medical geography of Rocky Mountain spotted fever in South Carolina, and Richard Parker's enthusiastic cooperation made it possible. I am particularly indebted to Logan Merritt for his ideas and assistance in developing approaches to understanding the geography of venereal disease in South Carolina.

This book was written for students and teachers of medical geography, and it is primarily directed toward those using it as a beginning basis for further explorations in spatial aspects of human health problems. There has never been a single-volume contribution in medical geography of sufficient scope to be used as a text for a course without supporting material, and I do not pretend that this book is an exception. I have attempted to establish a level of understanding suitable for advanced undergraduate and beginning graduate students. The book can be used best for a course in medical geography by considering each chapter as a central theme and expanding discussions with selected readings appropriate to the various topics.

The progression of logic from one chapter to the next ranges from ex-planations of basic concepts to the use of sophisticated research methods in medical geography. Throughout the book the importance of expectations of analytical results at different scales of geographical analysis is heavily emphasized. Since geography as a modern discipline has long since passed through a quantitative evolution in research methodologies, knowledge of basic statistics and simple concepts of spatial analysis are assumed on the part of the reader. If for some reason this is not the case, I recommend reading Peter Taylor's recent text on spatial analysis.

The first three chapters of the book are intended to be introductory in content and designed for the beginning student of medical geography. They should also serve as a review for more advanced scholars. The first chapter directs the reader to important contributions in medical geography over the past several decades within the context of conflict and survival in the environment. The second chapter is an explanation of how diseases are classified and transformed into measurable rates and ratios used in studies of medical geography. The third chapter addresses the topic of disease mapping at variable geographic scales. Emphasis in the third chapter is placed on methods and limitations of interpreting spatially derived disease patterns.

The next three chapters address methods used in determining reasons for variable spatial and temporal distributions of health problems. Chapter 4, on the subject of disease ecology, includes explanations of two recent North American health problems from a disease ecological point of view after an initial exposition of analytical methods used by medical geographers. The fifth chapter is an attempt to integrate geographical approaches used in the field of epidemiology with methods used by geographers in the study of spatial diffusion. Influenza is utilized as an example of how one might accomplish this integration. The sixth chapter addresses associative analysis in medical geography by discussing some statistical methods that have been used and suggesting a step-by-step procedure the medical geographer can follow in accomplishing comparisons.

The seventh and eighth chapters, along with a glossary of health planning terms, assist the reader in developing an understanding of how concepts of medical geography can be applied to planning for the provision of health care delivery services. Chapter 7 contains information explaining how methods of modern spatial analysis are used by the medical geographer as important ingredients in planning the location of future health care facilities. Aspects of optimal health care location models are then compared to the practical realities of the United States health care hierarchy, including economic and political barriers to more effective planning. Chapter 8 is a concise, straightforward explanation of how geographic base files can be used as important mechanisms for data acquisition by the medical geographer. The glossary of health planning terms was incorporated into this text to assist the reader in formulating a working knowledge of the many abbreviations and definitions incorporated into the bureaucratic process representing public policy in health planning. The student of medical geography intending to pursue a professional career as a health planner will find the latter inclusion particularly useful.

I have a few comments for my colleagues in medical geography who are actively pursuing these endeavors in theory and practice in the United States and many other countries. I am sure I omitted the important contributions of some, and this was by no means intentional. In developing this book my choices included: writing the book for the use of students more so than for highly advanced professional researchers; addressing a broad spectrum of international readers rather than a more limited number of North American medical geographers; assuming knowledge of modern methodologies of spatial analysis instead of developing a spatial-statistical treatise on human health problems; attempting to identify whenever possible how the results of studies in medical geography might be used to prevent human illness rather than constructing elaborate descriptive and "predictive" models only understood by those who have accomplished the same thing. Although this work will be used as a text for courses in medical geography it is also intended as a reference for many fellow geographers, health planners, allied health professionals, epidemiologists, and medical sociologists and anthropologists.

Sooner or later, writing a book places strains on family life. My deepest apologies to my wife, Carole, and my children, Eric and Frances, for periods of neglect. For the third time you have all inspired me to complete a book, and it would not have been possible without your assistance in so many ways.

Chapter 1

CONFLICT AND SURVIVAL IN ENVIRONMENTAL SYSTEMS

Man is an integral component of the ecological system of Planet Earth. As with other life forms within this system, the struggle for survival is based upon biological competition and/or co-existence. The phenomenon known as "life" is generated by chains of nucleoprotein—capable of nearly infinite adaptive modifications.[1] It is now known that nucleoprotein has been present since the beginnings of life, constantly operating on the principle of survival. From this "spark," all life has evolved in diverse forms ranging from magnificently beautiful to sometimes incredibly bizarre. In spite of size, shape and other identifying features, survival requires interaction with other nuclear protein in the form of food gathering, reproduction, and strengthening variations to ensure protection in the resultant conflict of living matter. Within a general biological context Man might be viewed as a miniscule component within chains of ecological survival systems. However, the development of cerebral powers has led to communications and hence collective efforts geared toward mutual protection. These efforts include protection against and control of disease.

Disease is best understood by most people within the context of health. Usually, disease does not preoccupy the majority of individuals when a state of "healthiness" exists. This is, in fact, what Cannon termed "homeostasis," and it implies a state of balance among multiple and diverse processes.[2] Disease is also a process, one which is manifested when this balance is somehow disrupted. Gordon developed a simple lever-fulcrum analogy to explain the impact environmental change or antigen mutation can have on disease agent and host (Man).[3] Within Gordon's system, biological balance exists when agent and host are at equilibrium (Figure 1). Changes in the nature of the agent, new strains of

1

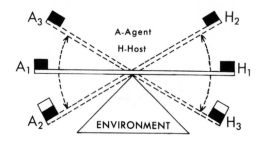

Fig. 1. An adaptation by Fox et al. of Gordon's analogy of agent–host relationships in states of balance and imbalance in the environment.

influenza, for example, can add weight to the agent (Position 2, Figure 1) and disrupt the balance. Conversely, Man as host can alter the environment in such a manner as to increase the susceptible population (Position 3). The optimum position of equilibrium within Gordon's scheme (Position 1) is a state of health.

Health and disease cannot be viewed as opposing sides of a coin but instead they are co-existing, overlapping states. Clearly, the ultimate disease damage to humans is death. Health is more difficult to define in an extreme sense because excellent health means far more than absence of illness. Philosophically, the World Health Organization (WHO) has defined "positive health" as the "state of complete physical, mental, and social well-being" and not merely the absence of disease or infirmity.[4] On the other hand, diseases represent "patterned responses or adaptations to harmful forces in the environment." In essence, disease can be defined in a general sense as some form of departure from a state of health resulting from dysfunction of homeostatic mechanisms—a consequence of imbalance with environment (social, biological, physiological).

In understanding health as a state, the terms "functioning," "adapting," and "normal" are important. Environment broadly defined includes state of health in terms of kind of environment, kind of stimuli within the particular environment(s) and response to stimuli within the environment(s). Dolfman offers the following operational definition of health:[5]

> An individual is healthy (that is, has attained or is in the state or condition known as health) if he is functioning adequately in a stated environment; and if while functioning in this environment he is subjected to some sort of stress, he is able to adapt to this stress within the range of normal functioning.

> Conversely,

> An individual is not healthy if he is not functioning adequately in a stated environment; or if while functioning in this environment, he is subjected to some sort of stress, he does not adapt within the range of normal functioning.

Clearly, geographers have been concerned, indeed, even preoccupied with environmental problems for centuries. Modern definitions of environment encompass a wide range of social and cultural conditions as well as more traditional natural habitats.[6] The study of spatial aspects of disease and health care are logical extensions of trends in geographical analysis that have developed during this century. Within these contexts, health problems are viewed as environmental problems requiring the use of spatial research techniques to assist in understanding and, in some instances, explanation.

ESSENTIALS OF MEDICAL GEOGRAPHY

The term "medical geography" has different meanings to different people. The idea of studying the geography of disease can in some respects be interpreted as a narrow subfield of either medicine or geography. In reality, medical geography is a multidimensional body of knowledge and at the same time a multifaceted approach geared toward understanding spatial aspects of human health problems.[7] A wide variety of natural and social scientific methods must be utilized and/or developed to comprehensively accomplish such studies. Writers taking various topical approaches to medical geography quite often study relationships between natural environment and contagious disease (disease ecology), while others develop various methodologies for detailed mapping of disease patterns to the ends that singular or multiple associations with cultural and naturally occurring phenomena can be identified and perhaps better understood. Some researchers produce analyses of the geographical spread, or, diffusion of diseases from endemic foci to other places in time and space, while yet other spatial studies of human health problems deal with the administration and provision of treatment facilities. These and many other topical approaches can add much to our knowledge of human health conditions. However, a holistic understanding of the essence of medical geography is not necessarily to be found by exploration of the variety of topical approaches, particularly if any are taken in deterministic isolation. If applications are to be meaningful, it is first necessary to develop an understanding of the conceptual basis of medical geography. This basis is not static, and it has grown and become increasingly complex. As a result, the interaction among naturally occurring and man-made phenomena in relation to health problems has become more clearly understandable. It is thus suggested here that an understanding of medical geography is best developed and understood within an evolutionary context.

It is not difficult to encounter reconstructions of epidemics in history written for popular consumption. Many such works frequently make reference to the Greeks as having first developed an understanding of the importance of geographical variations of health problems. Other references can be found to the works of the Arabs during the European Dark Ages. This literature on disease in history has added to our knowledge of disease-specific environments. In addition, modern medical knowledge has assisted in explaining such problems as the diffusion of plague in Europe in the 1300s as well as many ailments of earlier societies. Maps are frequently used in such studies to explain general patterns of distribution in relation to social and economic conditions as well as perceptions of local populations and are often followed by up-to-date reactions in light of improved scientific knowledge. With the exception of the contributions of Melvyn Howe,[8] few researchers have gone beyond the mere descriptive to search for more serious considerations of the multiplicity of geographical factors involved. This often results in sound historical research becoming clouded by romantic notions creating protective barriers for our modern Western culture in particular.

Various accounts written during the 18th and 19th centuries dwelled on geographical influences of disease. Some identified specific outbreaks of contagious diseases within cities and others rendered accounts of exotic ailments endemic to distant locations. Still, knowledge of the diffusion of disease in conjunction with improved communications networks helped contribute to the international public health movement in the 19th century. This era of research was crowned by the classic efforts of August Hirsch in the development of a three-volume handbook of historical and geographical pathology.[9] Such studies nearly come to a halt, however, as a result of microbiologic breakthroughs and the identification of specific disease-causing elements.

Geographic studies of disease at the end of the 19th and beginning of the 20th centuries could be viewed as a tradition of separate writers addressing analyses of single diseases. As knowledge of agents causing contagious diseases grew, so did these kinds of studies. During the first part of the 20th century, a plethora of works loosely termed medical geography were produced, particularly in Western Europe and the United States; although the geographic areas covered included most parts of the world.[10] The major emphasis of these studies was the impact of the environment on human health conditions with particular emphasis on climate. Examples of this orientation included the works of Earl Baldwin McKinley and James Stevens Simmons. McKinley's studies resulted from questionnaire findings in the early 1930s wherein diseases were classified in accordance with tropical and temperate climates.[11] The three volumes produced by Simmons consisted of a country-by-country inventory of diseases in parts of the world where human contacts with natural environmental elements are the most frequent.[12]

As the environmentally oriented approaches were in keeping with developments of epidemiology and public health, so were studies geared toward understanding disease problems in more industrialized parts of the world. Social and cultural differences were taken as determinants of the spatial variability of disease and ill health in industrialized nations.[13] In geographic scale, the approach was implied to have worldwide implications, but many findings were based on local and urban analyses. The contents of many of these contributions generally included the identification of maladies particular to cultural or subcultural groups. For example, an early view of York, England by B. S. Rowntree at the end of the 19th century placed a great deal of emphasis on poverty as a determinant of health conditions.[14] Rowntree described "unsanitary" conditions in quarters of lower class industrial workers, attempting to vividly depict the potential for breeding of disease agents in relation to dwelling conditions. One method used by Rowntree in reaching such conclusions was the comparison of groups of school children and British army applicants from poverty areas, finding both groups smaller in height than their counterparts from other areas.

During the Second World War and the period immediately following, medical geographers continued to place particular emphasis on environmental factors and distribution of disease—and for good reasons. Opposing troops during World War II in many parts of the world were exposed to a myriad of disease-producing agents. As an outgrowth of German efforts, the *World Atlas of Epidemic Diseases* by Rodenwaldt and Jusatz was brought to fruition during the pre-World War II period with assistance from the United States Navy.[15] The works of Rodenwaldt and Jusatz were monumental in comparison to previous attempts to define environmentally-oriented diseases, and the three volume work is still utilized as a reference in terms of environmental risk factors for many diseases.

In 1950 the American Geographical Society brought Jacques M. May, the French medical geographer, to the United States with the avowed aim of developing an atlas of disease in keeping with current geographical thinking in this subject area.[16] May accomplished a good deal more than the production of a simple atlas. While the atlas was released in sheet form over a five-year period (until 1955), May also wrote articles revolving around his concepts of two-, three-, and four-factor host-environment-reservoir relationships. May further defined disease ecology.[17] The concept of disease ecology is more epidemiologically oriented than many approaches to medical geography.[18] Disease ecology is explained in more detail in Chapter 4, emphasizing that environment, particularly climate, can become an overriding factor in the understanding of human disease problems.

In North America, the three decades following the Second World War witnessed the development of a wider variety of comprehensive studies in the area of medical geography than had been accomplished for centuries before. This is somewhat incredible in light of the notion of Ackernecht that, "by 1940 the very concept of a geography of diseases had been virtually erased from the memory of the practicing physician."[19] In other words, primarily due to the advent of such "miracle" drugs as penicillin, Aureomycin, and Terramycin, many medical practitioners no longer felt the need to be concerned with geographic aspects of environmental risk factors. On the other hand, professionally trained geographers were synthesizing many notions that had been developed over the years by public health workers, epidemiologists and other nongeographers. Such a movement paralleled what has been considered the culmination of repeated international efforts geared toward the standardization of disease classification systems (international disease classification developments are discussed in Chapter 2).

Given the emphasis of many pioneer researchers in medical geography on the examination of disease distributions from an international perspective, it is important to understand the ramifications and limitations of major conclusions which have been and continue to be drawn. In spite of the continued diffusion of modern medical technology throughout the world, concepts of disease and disease treatment understood as part of Western culture are not necessarily in keeping with concepts of health and disease in many other parts of the world. The most striking example is the traditional Chinese philosophy of health and disease treatment in contrast to recent developments in the area of preventive medical care.[20] In addition, pluralistic or folk and modern disease treatment measures are still practiced simultaneously in much of the Third World.[21] Even within Western and industrial nations, scientific training in various health-related disciplines, as well as within different countries and specific subcultures, varies considerably. Differing degrees of economic development as well as social and political institutional differences have also had some bearing on scientific training as well as resultant approaches to understanding medical geography. Also, past and present international spheres of political and economic influence throughout the world often influence the direction of research in medical geography.

If there is truly an "international" effort to understand the geography of disease, it is reflected in the efforts of the WHO and the United Nations. WHO, actually a semi-independent foundation of the United Nations, has followed, through the use of expert committees, the more traditional epidemiological approach of supporting clinically-oriented case studies of disease problems in specific locations. While WHO support of research in medical geography has been on a somewhat limited basis, analyses of disease in relation to biological, chemical, climatic and other environmental elements have been completed in a gross manner. Also, some geographical conclusions keep on being made from WHO-supported health care delivery services provided to specified locations throughout the world as well as from recommendations WHO has made for environmental controls projected as solutions to health problems. Information useful to international medicogeographical research is provided by WHO in various forms. National disease specific mortality rates based on periodic revision of the International Disease Classification System are published annually in United Nations demographic yearbooks. The results of various studies and programs to alleviate malnutrition and to provide more modern medical treatment facilities in different parts of the world often provide geographic data. Limitations to truly comprehensive international research include the lack of annual reporting from many countries, including the Soviet Union, mainland China and many Third World countries, as well as the more microscale clinical approach utilized in WHO-sponsored epidemiological research. This situation does not preclude the accomplishment of international comparisons; however, it should be understood that conclusions made from analytical results of spatial comparisons are restricted to knowledge of disease problems in countries voluntarily reporting to the WHO.

Within the more narrow confines of the discipline of geography, national educational systems have influenced what might be termed particular types of national or perhaps supranational efforts in the area of medical geography. For example, within Britain and some former commonwealth countries several clearly identifiable trends in medical geography have been brought to fruition since World War II. Such major schools of thought include the perfection of techniques in mapping disease and health problems, associative studies, i.e., comparing cartographic patterns with the distribution of factors related to health problems, disease diffusion and studies of the ecology of health, including both natural and man-made environments. Andrew Learmonth's now classic studies of geographic factors contributing to the ecology of malaria in India, as well as his more recent contribution pertaining to the geography of hunger, exemplify some of the British trends.[22] Melvin Howe's monumental contributions in the area of disease mapping have shown how some simple to more complex variations in cartographic techniques may lead to variable interpretations of health problems.[23] Neil McGlashan has further brought disease mapping closer to a fine art by augmenting traditional methods of probabilistic mapping with simultaneous epidemiological associations.[24] In the area of disease diffusion, R. Mansell Prothero and Arthur Brownlea have respectively shown how malaria has diffused with migration and how hepatitis can be identified as following patterns of human settlement growth.[25] In fact, from its onset in 1949 to its termination in 1976, the Commission on Medical Geography of the International Geographical Union was clearly dominated by British approaches. If there is indeed a single "commonwealth" approach to medical geography, its main strengths are in the areas of disease mapping and regional synthesis of health problems.

Efforts in the area of medical geography in Germany, Japan, and Belgium demonstrate certain trends parallel to those in Britain, but with varying degrees of uniqueness. In Germany, Helmut Jusatz, a pioneer researcher in medical geography and one of the major authors of the *Welt-Seuchen Atlas* has continued to offer direction in the areas of medical cartography and geographical pathology.[26] Momiyama has shown how climate and the subsequent effects of modernization in Japan have influenced the seasonality of mortality for several decades.[27] Recent studies of the international geography of cancer, developed under the leadership of Yola Verhasselt of Brussels, have gained international recognition.[28]

In France, the foundations of medical geography for several decades were based on the many works of Max Sorre. He undertook a variety of local studies, and is best known internationally for his concepts of human ecology of space inhabited by man.[29] His major contributions in the area of medical geography included studies of climate and man, human nutrition and the human organism struggling against the natural environment. Recently, Henri Picheral has taken a new approach to medical geography in France via his regional, and, to some extent, cartographic analyses of socioeconomic influences of health problems in the Midi Mediterranean.[30]

Soviet scientists, no doubt due to the harsh environment of many parts of the U.S.S.R., have long been concerned with biogeographic aspects of medical geography. According to Markovin in a documentation of the history of the development of medical geography within the Soviet Union, concerns about the environment can be traced to early Russian chronicles in the 15th century.[31] The first Soviet conference on problems in medical geography was held in Leningrad in 1962.[32] During that conference the five major problems in medical geography discussed included: (1) methodologies in medical geography and the education of medical geographers; (2) medicogeographical analyses of natural territorial complexes; (3) regional medical geography studies within the Soviet Union as well as other countries; (4) the study of the geographical distribution of diseases (nosogeography); and (5) medical-geographic mapping. By the mid-1960s, Yevgeiniy I. Ignatyev and his associates defined medical geography as the study of the spatial distribution of health, illness, and diseases that can essentially be grouped into three major categories.[33] The categories included the analysis of the distribution of human diseases and contributing conditions, the effects of natural conditions on health, and the analysis of geographical environments and their influence on health. As with many systems of scientific classification, these three general categories demonstrate a degree of overlap in approach. In 1976, Voronov continued to reiterate the views of most Soviet medical geographers that, aside from some diseases which appear to be of hereditary origin, studies in medical geography should be primarily concerned with environmental risk factors.[34] Medical geography in the Soviet Union is highly centralized and most efforts are now directed through the Medical Geography Laboratory of the Department of Biogeography at Moscow University.

Within the United States and Canada, concurrent approaches to medical geography have emerged since the Second World War. The influence of Jacques May is still paramount, and North American medical geographers continue to carry on field studies in various environments in attempts to either corroborate past findings or offer new evidence in the area of disease ecology. In addition, Armstrong and Meade have added important cultural ingredients to such approaches.[35] Disease mapping has continued to be an important trend. Earlier methodological statements in this area were put forth by Malcolm Murray, and by the late 1970s federal agencies in the United States had begun to incorporate various types of disease mapping in published reports.[36] Other North American researchers have combined principles of epidemiology, disease ecology and the mapping of disease into analyses helping to explain processes in the spatial diffusion of health problems (these works are discussed at length in Chapter 5). While by no means unique to the United States, a major trend in the general area of medical geography deals with spatial aspects of the provision of health services and the allocation of facilities. Part of this latter trend is due to the role geographers have played in the overall process of health planning, but the trend has also been influenced by geographic evidence of the peculiarities of the American health care delivery system resulting from the overall lack of comprehensive national policy.[35]

Regardless of the continued probability of national or supranational research trends because of the reasons mentioned above, several specific methodological statements on the nature of medical geography have been put forth. For many analyses, May's logic of 1950 may be as appropriate now as when he put forth the notion that disease is a multiple phenomena occurring only when various factors coincide in time and space. The focus of interest widens to encompass the relationships identified among a variety of factors of this complex and their respective geographic environments. More recently, John Hunter expanded upon May's concept with the following statement, "The application of geographical concepts and techniques to health-related problems" can be called medical geography.[38] In defining environment, Hunter included physical, biological, social, cultural and economic components. McGlashan has made several statements about the nature of medical geography, primarily with emphasis on communication with the medical profession. In general, McGlashan has contended that it is the role of the geographer to explain where diseases are occurring and to support these occurrences with geographical correlates.[39] McGlashan further contends that while the geographer may not offer proof to the medical practitioner, there is certainly the possibility of offering evidence.[40]

Medical geography is, or can be, the spatial analysis of most aspects of human health problems. So long as there are geographic variations in time and space, whether related to naturally occurring or artificial environments (We must also realize that environments change over time), there is a definite need for geographic applications and communication of research findings. Perhaps more than some other discipline, geography periodically tends to become introspective. Yet medical geography must be interdisciplinary by its very nature.[41] Furthermore, medical geography has evolved over time, particularly within the last two decades. Medical geography has changed during that time period in a fashion similar to the discipline of geography in general, particularly because it has been receiving continued influences from a variety of approaches utilized by many scientific disciplines. The result is conceptual overlap. Depending upon the subject matter under investigation, as well as the orientation of the researcher, various spatial approaches are required. Figure 2 is intended to show the overlap of some of these approaches and how they might change over time. For example, approaching a study in medical geography from an environmental point of view requires some overlap, when the information is possible, with information about genetic aspects of human health as well as human behavior, the epidemiology of

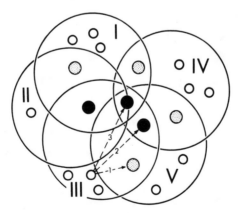

VARIOUS SPATIAL APPROACHES

I. Environmental II. Genetic III. Epidemiological IV. Behavioral V. Socioeconomic

Fig. 2. An example of various conceptual approaches to the study of medical geography.

particular diseases and socioeconomic conditions. At a point in time, the study of an infectious disease may be primarily due to epidemiological determinants. However, as shown within Figure 2, at another point in time socioeconomic conditions should also be brought into play. At yet additional times the researcher must also consider human behavior or perhaps ultimately all of the approaches shown within the illustration to develop a truly holistic understanding of spatial aspects of the health problem.

When geographic scale is added to various approaches as a necessary ingredient of medical geography, concepts of definition become even more complex. An examination of the medical geography literature shows that particular combinations of approach and scale have been utilized to a major or minor degree by different researchers.[42] These combinations have been diagrammed within Figure 3. In approaches intended to demonstrate disease mapping, for example, most such studies have focused at the national level. Medical geography studies utilizing either a disease ecological or a cultural ecological approach have been basically either international, national, or regional; however, some studies of these natures have been aspatial. Again, because of the availability of information, studies in the diffusion of disease have been primarily national, with some emphasis on international, regional and interurban scales. By contrast, studies of disease association have been more prominent at the regional,

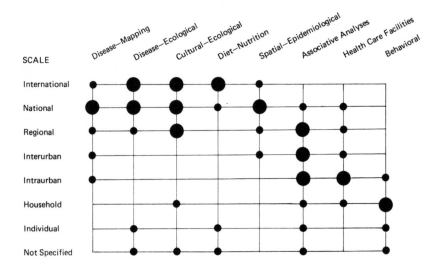

Fig. 3. General topical approaches to medical geography compared with different geographic scales. Large black dots indicate where most attention has been paid by writings in medical geography and the smaller black dots are intended to show where lesser attention has been given.

interurban and intraurban scales. Studies pertaining to the geography of health care have been predominantly intraurban, but some research has been done at the interurban and national scales as well as the household level. Aspects of behavior in medical geography, while limited in volume, have been the most successful at the household level. This cross-tabulation of approaches by geographic scale is not intended as an agenda necessarily for research in medical geography. Nonetheless, some of the constraints mentioned in this chapter appear to be controlling the direction of approaches to medical geography in relation to geographic scale. The remainder of this book is devoted to offering specific examples of some of these approaches to medical geography. In the process the various geographic scales operate either advantageously or as constraints to the results.

NOTES

[1] Fraser Brockington. *World Health*. Edinburgh: Churchill Livingston (1975), pp. 8–12.

[2] Walter B. Cannon. *The Wisdom of the Body*. New York: W. W. Norton (1932).

[3] This concept is discussed in John P. Fox, Carrie E. Hall and Lila R. Elveback. *Epidemiology, Man and Disease*. London: Macmillan (1970), pp. 34–36. Also see J. E. Gordon and T. H. Ingalls. "Medical Ecology and the Public Health," *American Journal of Medical Science*, Vol. 235 (1958), pp. 337–359.

[4] Brockington, op. cit., pp. 1–7.

[5] Michael L. Dolfman. "Toward Operational Definitions of Health," *The Journal of School Health*, Vol. 64 (1974), pp. 206–209.

[6] Marvin W. Mikesell. "Geography as the Study of Environment: An Assessment of Some Old and New Commitments" in Ian R. Manners and Marvin W. Mikesell (eds.). *Perspectives on Environment*. Washington: Association of American Geographers (1974), pp. 1–23.

[7] Gerald F. Pyle. "International Communication and Medical Geography," *Social Science and Medicine*, Vol. 11 (1977), pp. 1–4.

[8] G. Melvyn Howe. *Man, Environment and Disease in Britain*. New York: Barns and Noble (1972).

[9] August Hirsch. *Handbook of Geographical and Historical Pathology* (3 vols.). London: New Sydenham Society (1883–1886).

[10] Albert P. Bright. "Problems of Geographic Influence," *Annals*, Association of American Geographers, Vol. 15 (1915).

[11] Earl Baldwin McKinley. *A Geography of Disease*. Washington: George Washington University Press (1935).

[12] James Stevens Simmons, et al. *Global Epidemiology* (3 vols.). Philadelphia: J. B. Lippincott (1944–1954).

[13] A. Leslie Banks. "The Study of Geography of Disease," *Geographical Journal*, Vol. 125 (1959), pp. 199–210.

[14] B. Seebohm Rowntree. *Poverty, A Study of Town Life*. London: Macmillan (1901), pp. 182–221.

[15] Ernst Rodenwaldt and Helmut J. Jusatz (eds.). *Welt-Seuchen-Atlas* (World Atlas of Epidemic Diseases). 3 vols. published in German and English. Hamburg: Falk (1952–1961).

[16] R. U. Light. "The Progress of Medical Geography," *Geographical Review*, Vol. 34 (1944), pp. 36–41.

[17] Jacques M. May. *Studies in Disease Ecology*. New York: Hafner Publishing Co. (1961). From 1950–1955 the American Geographical Society of New York featured 17 published streets of the *Atlas of Diseases* in various issues of *Geographical Review*. They are listed by title and number: World Distribution of Poliomyelitis, 1900–1950, Vol. 40 (October, 1950), 648–49; World Distribution of Cholera, 1816–1950, Vol. 41 (April, 1951), 272–73; World Distribution of Malaria Vectors, Vol. 41 (October, 1951), 638–39; World Distribution of Helminthiases, Vol. 41 (January, 1952), 98–101; World Distribution of Dengue and Yellow Fever, Vol. 42 (April, 1952), 282–83; World Distribution of Plague, Vol. 42 (October, 1952), 628–30; World Distribution of Leprosy, Vol. 43 (January, 1953), 89–90; Study in Human Starvation, 1. Sources of Selected Foods, Vol. 43 (April, 1953), 253–55; and Study in Human Starvation, 2. Diets and Deficiency Diseases, Vol. 43 (July, 1953), 404–4. World Distribution of Rickettsial Diseases: Louse-borne and Flea-borne Typhus, Vol. 44 (January, 1954), 133–36; Tick-borne and Mite-borne Forms, Vol. 44 (January, 1954), 133–36; Tick and Mite Vectors, Vol. 44 (April, 1954), 133–36; Explored Areas of Arthropod-borne Viral Infections (excl. Yellow Fever and Dengue), Vol. 44 (July, 1954), 408–10; and World Distribution of Leishmaniases, Vol. 44 (October, 1954), 583–84. World Distribution of Spirochetal Diseases: World Distribution of Yaws, Vol. 45 (July, 1955), 416; Louse-borne and Tick-borne, Vol. 45 (October, 1955), 572; and Leptospiroses, Vol. 45 (October, 1955), 572.

[18] Jacques M. May. *The Etiology of Human Disease*. New York: M.D. Publications (1958).

[19] E. H. Ackernecht. *History and Geography of the Most Important Diseases*. New York: Hafner (1965).

[20] Katherine Gould-Martin. "Hot Cold Clean Poison and Dirt: Chinese Folk Medical Categories," *Social Science and Medicine*, Vol. 12, No. 1B (January, 1978), pp. 39–46.

[21] Charles M. Good. "Traditional Medicine: An Agenda for Medical Geography," *Social Science and Medicine*, Vol. 11, No. 14–16 (November, 1977), pp. 705–713.

[22] A. T. A. Learmonth. "Medical Geography in India and Pakistan," *Geographical Journal*, Vol. 127 (1961), pp. 10–26.

[23] G. Melvyn Howe. *National Atlas of Disease Mortality in the United Kingdom (1954-58)*. London: Nelson (1963).

[24] Neil McGlashan. "Uses of the Poisson Probability Model with Human Populations," *Pacific Viewpoint*, Vol. 17 (1976), pp. 167–174.

[25] See R. Mansell Prothero. *Migrants and Malaria*. London: Longmans (1965). A. A. Brownlea. "An Urban Ecology of Infectious Disease: City of Greater Wollongong-Shell Harbour," *Australian Geographer*, Vol. 10 (1967), pp. 169–187.

[26] H. J. Jusatz. "Zur Entwicklungsgeschichte der medizinisch-geographischen Karten in Deutschland," *Mitteilungen der Reichsamps für Landesaufnahme*, No. 1 (1939), pp. 11–22; "Aufgaben and Methoden der Medizinschen Kartographie," *Petermans Geographische Mitteilungen*, Vol. 90 (1944), pp. 219–225; and "Fortschritte der Medizinsche Kargographie," *Petermans Geographische Mitteilungen*, Vol. 101 (1957), pp. 304–306.

[27] Masako Sakamoto-Momiyama. *Seasonality in Human Mortality*. Tokyo: University of Tokyo Press (1977).

[28] Vola Verhasselt. *Maps on Cancer Distribution*. Brussels: Vrije Universiteit Brussel, Geografisch Instituut (1975).

[29] Maximilien Sorre. "Principes Généraux de la Géographie Médicale," in *Fondements Biologiques de la Géographie Humaine* (1943). Reprinted in Paris in 1971 by Arnard Colin.

[30] Henri Picheral. *Espace et Santé: Géographie Médicale du Midi de la France*. Montepellier: Inprimerie du "Paysan du Midi" (1976).

[31] A. P. Markovin. "Historical Sketch of the Development of Soviet Medical Geography," *Soviet Geography*, Vol. 3 (1962), pp. 3–19.

[32] O. V. Shkurlatov, "The First Soviet Conference on Problems in Medical Geography," *Soviet Geography,* Vol. 4 (1963), pp. 55–57.

[33] T. M. Gelyakova, A. G. Voronov, V. B. Nefedova, and G. S. Samoylova. "The Present State of Medical Geography in the U.S.S.R.," *Soviet Geography,* Vol. 8 (1967), pp. 228–234. Also see Razia Khan. "Purpose, Scope and Progress of Medical Geography," *Indian Geographical Journal,* Vol. 46 (1971), pp. 1–9. A. V. Chaklin. "The Geographical Distribution of Cancer in the Soviet Union," *Soviet Geography,* Vol. 3 (1962), pp. 59–68.

[34] A. G. Voronov, "The Geographical Environment and Human Health," *Soviet Geography,* Vol. 18 (1977), pp. 230–237.

[35] R. W. Armstrong. "The Geography of Specific Environments of Patients and Non-Patients in Cancer Studies, with a Malaysian Example," *Economic Geography,* Vol. 52 (1976), pp. 161–170. Melinda Meade. "Land Development and Human Health in West Malaysia," *Annals,* Association of American Geographers, Vol. 66 (1976), pp. 428–439.

[36] Malcolm A. Murray. "Geography of Death in the United States and the United Kingdom," *Annals,* Association of American Geographers, Vol. 58 (1967), pp. 301–315.

[37] Gary W. Shannon and G. E. Alan Dever. *Health Care Delivery: Spatial Perspectives.* New York: McGraw–Hill (1974).

[38] John M. Hunter. "The Challenge of Medical Geography," *The Geography of Health and Disease.* Chapel Hill, North Carolina: Department of Geography, University of North Carolina (1974).

[39] N. D. McGlashan. "The Scope of Medical Geography," *South African Geographical Journal,* Vol. 47 (1965), pp. 35–40, and "The Medical Geographer's Work," *International Pathology,* Vol. 7 (1966), pp. 81–83.

[40] N. D. McGlashan. "Geographical Evidence on Medical Hypotheses," *Tropical and Geographical Medicine,* Vol. 19 (1967), pp. 333–343.

[41] Gerald F. Pyle. "Introduction: Foundations to Medical Geography," *Economic Geography,* Vol. 52 (1976), pp. 95–102.

[42] Gerald F. Pyle, op. cit.

Chapter 2

DISEASE CLASSIFICATION AND MEASUREMENT SYSTEMS

General knowledge of disease classification and measurement systems is essential to understanding the various intersecting approaches to medical geography. These systems have also grown in an overlapping fashion and can now be considered the results of several historical trends. Scholars of the history of medicine have written about state doctors in ancient Egypt and of the societal controls initiated by the Greeks.[1] We know of the works of Galen in the area of hygiene in Rome in the second century A.D. Other accounts explain the leprosaria of the Middle Ages, the quarantine movement which started in Venice, sanitary inspectors in Cordoba and other Arab cities, and of embryonic municipal public health movements initially spurred by the Renaissance.[2] By the late seventeenth and into the eighteenth centuries, knowledge of many causes of human illness and disease control measures were beginning to increase. Variable European developments in the area of social medicine led to the public health movement.[3] Both physiological and social approaches to disease control depended primarily upon knowledge of precisely what to measure and subsequently spurred the development of systems of disease accounting, or, how to measure.

With what is now considered minimal knowledge of disease etiology and with no strong early attempts to coalesce apparent causes of death with morbidity, striking contributions in the area of measurement were made. For example, William Petty, the pioneer political arithmetician, espoused the ideas of John Graunt and put forth the notion that health needs of a population should be surveyed, and these needs should be compared with an inventory of medical practitioners and facilities.[4] In Germany, the Cameralist approach to social problems was strongly supported by Veit Ludwig von Secendorf in the organization and administration of *Medizinalpolizei* (Medical Police). Efforts in the area of implementing medical police are reflected in the works of Johann Peter Frank, a pioneer worker in public health. Frank's works (*Medicinische Polizei*), published from 1822 to 1827, had a strong influence on many continental European programs as well as eventually some in Great Britain and the United States.[5] Related public health control programs developed particularly in Britain as a result of the contributions of Edwin Chadwick on health and sanitation. Particular emphasis was placed on improved drainage and water purification.

By the middle of the nineteenth century, and this was prior to major discoveries of most disease-causing agents, hygiene and sanitation programs had been put into effect in many industrial nations. William Farr put forth an argument for standardized disease tables, with the intent to codify morbidity and mortality. However, while some discoveries had been made, for example, Jenner's discovery in 1798 of cowpox vaccination for smallpox, there was still insufficient cooperation among public authorities attempting to control and quarantine epidemics and many medical practitioners. Still, in 1851 the first major international conference on sanitation was held in Paris.[6] No less than nine more meetings were held in 1897 in different major world cities. Quite often the major topics of these conferences were particular diseases, for example, cholera or plague.

By the beginning of the twentieth century many important biological discoveries had been made, and, while they were not always accepted by established medical groups immediately, an eventual understanding of these processes became more widely accepted. Pasteur, along with many of his other contributions, had given us preventive measures for hydrophobia in 1885.[7] In 1884, Robert Koch had identified the cholera bacillus, and the cause of tuberculosis was also uncovered. There was knowledge that the plague was somehow related to rat populations, yellow fever to mosquitos, and typhus to lice.

In 1907, as a result of an international sanitary conference held in Paris several years earlier, an international office of public health known as the *Office International d'Hygiene Publique* (OIHP) was established. The main function of the OIHP was to disseminate to member states information about health-related matters, particularly about such communicable diseases as cholera, plague, and yellow fever. The OIHP thus became the first modern international disease control headquarters. In order to accomplish any forms of disease control it was necessary to adopt methods of standardized disease classification for purposes of information dissemination and similar functions. By 1923, the functions of the OIHP had been absorbed by the League of Nations Health Organization. Early work of the latter organization was primarily directed toward some of the health problems which had surfaced (or resurfaced in some instances) during World War I and epidemics which had diffused during the early 1920s. In addition, some important research was supported by the health organization of the League pertaining to such chronic ailments as cancer. Yet further accomplishments in social and economic illness associations have also been recorded. By the time World War II had begun, the fifth revision (1938) of the *International*

Classification of Diseases was in use in many parts of the world. The scientific and technological developments emanating from World War II were carried into our knowledge of specific diseases. This knowledge was of considerable importance when a world attempting to rebuild peace sent delegates to form the United Nations with a single health organization. By 1948, the World Health Organization was created after several years of planning and development. WHO then assumed many functions of the earlier international health organizations and succeeded in integrating several regional health groups. Since then efforts toward biological standardization and categorical redefinition have been included in subsequent revisions of the *International Classification of Diseases.* In general, the taxonomic philosophy of the system is to divide causes of death into broad groups. The classification first deals with diseases caused by infective agents, followed by categories for cancers, allergic disorders, and then nutritional deficiencies. In addition, such aspects as congenital deficiencies, mental illness problems and those due to accidents have been incorporated. The eighth revision, developed in 1965, added some refinements to this system. An abbreviated list of the eighth revision of major causes of death is included here as Table 1. International plans are now underway for yet another revision of the *International Classification of Diseases.* At the time of this writing, the ninth revision (1975: published 1977) is just being adopted.

CAUSAL FACTORS IN HUMAN ILLNESS

The momentum that has built up over the past centuries in search of more and more knowledge about causal factors in human illness will no doubt continue. Periodic revisions of the international disease classification system are one manifestation of the depth and direction of such efforts. In fact, the quest for contributory causes of human illness and death is so complex that it has been described as endless.[8] Generally termed *etiology* (From Greek, *aitia,* or cause), the analysis of causes of disease and death has greatly influenced our methods of classifying health problems. In some instances, initiating agents are considered pathological factors or *pathogens.* For example, several types of viruses are known to be primary agents that attack human systems and cause influenza. Manifestations, or signs (readily discernible) and symptoms (not always apparent) lead to diagnosis of the disease and usually the agent. For example, termed *morbidity,* the illness condition, influenza, can be traced to a viral agent; however, complications leading to pneumonic conditions subsequently causing death (*mortality*) result in an "influenza–pneumonia" cause of death rubric. Yet pneumonia may be caused by different kinds of organisms, and it is serious and life-threating to the very young, the elderly, and to others with higher levels of susceptibility—for one reason or another.

In spite of knowledge of the possibility of multiple-causality in illness, there is still a tendency on the part of many diagnosticians to quickly arrive at single causes of disease and etiology. Conversely, it is common practice to identify a *primary* cause of either morbidity or mortality. These primary causes are directly

Table 1. List of 50 Causes for Tabulation of Mortality

Cause groups	Detailed list numbers	Cause groups	Detailed list numbers
B 1 Cholera	000	B33 Bronchitis, emphysema and asthma	490–493
B 2 Typhoid Fever	001	B34 Peptic ulcer	531–533
B 3 Bacillary dysentery and amoebiasis	004, 006	B35 Appendicitis	540–543
B 4 Enteritis and other diarrhoeal diseases	008, 009	B36 Intestinal obstruction and hernia	(550–553 / 560
B 5 Tuberculosis of respiratory system	010–012	B37 Cirrhosis of liver	571
B 6 Other tuberculosis, including late effects	013–019	B38 Nephritis and nephrosis	580–584
B 7 Plague	020	B39 Hyperplasia of prostate	600
B 8 Diphtheria	032	B40 Abortion	640–645
B 9 Whooping cough	033	B41 Other complications of pregnancy, childbirth and the puerperium. Delivery without mention of complications.	(631–639 / 659–678
B10 Streptococcal sore throat and scarlet fever	034	B42 Congenital anomalies	740–759
B11 Meningococcal infection	036	B43 Birth injury, difficult labour and other anoxic and hypoxic conditions.	(764–768 / 772, 776
B12 Acute poliomyelitis	040–043	B44 Other causes of perinatal mortality	(769–771 / 773–775 / 777–779
B13 Smallpox	050	B45 Symptoms and ill-defined conditions	780–796
B14 Measles	055	B46 All other diseases	(Remainder of 240–738
B15 Typhus and other rickettsioses	080–083	External Cause of Injury	
B16 Malaria	084	BE47 Motor vehicle accidents	E810–E823
B17 Syphillis and its sequelae	090–097	BE48 All other accidents	(E800–E807 / E825–E949
B18 All other infective and parasitic diseases	(Remainder of 000–136	BE49 Suicide and self-inflicted injuries	E950–959E
B19 Malignant neoplasms, including neoplasms of lymphatic and haematopoietic tissue	140–209	BE50 All other external causes	E960–E999
B20 Benign neoplasms and neoplasms of unspecified nature	210–239	Nature of Injury	
B21 Diabetes mellitus	250	BN47 Fractures, intracranial and internal injuries	(N800–N828 / N850–N869
B22 Avitaminoses and other nutritional deficiency	260–269	BN48 Burn	N940–N949
B23 Anaemias	280–285	BN49 Adverse effects of chemical substances	N960–N989
B24 Meningitis	320	BN50 All other injuries	(Remainder of N800–N999
B25 Active rheumatic fever	390–392		
B26 Chronic rheumatic heart disease	393–398		
B27 Hypertensive disease	400–404		
B28 Ischaemic heart disease	410–414		
B29 Other forms of heart disease	420–429		
B30 Cerebrovascular disease	430–438		
B31 Influenza	470–474		
B32 Pneumonia	480–486		

Source: Manual of the International Statistical Classification of Diseases, Injuries, and Causes of Death, Vol. 1, Geneva: World Health Organization, 1967 (8th Revision).

linked to environmental systems. Furthermore, generalized *infectious* and *chronic* cycles of disease patterns have been identified. Dever has explained these cycles within the contexts of an agrarian cultural influence (environments producing infectious disease problems) and chronic diseases more common to industrial and post-industrial societies.[9] Infectious and chronic disease cycles are depicted within Figure 4. Developing nations and even some rural parts of developed nations are often characterized by more harsh environments interacting with higher fertility, infectious and parasitic diseases, malnutrition and high mortality risks for the very young. More industrialized and economically developed societies are conversely afflicted by a range of chronic diseases.

Infectious Diseases

Perhaps as much as two-thirds of all human illness can be attributed to microorganisms concerned with their own biological survival in human tissue. The human body offers favorable conditions for the multiplication of these parasites living in susceptible cells. As explained by Burton and Smith:[10]

> For the parasite to affect the host fatally is not usually the most successful result, as the infecting agent may perish with the host. Long continued association of parasite with a host population results in the evolution of a biological balance, satisfactory to the parasite and generally tolerable to the host.

Favorable multiplication in turn leads to transfer to another host. Much of the time parasites have the ability to colonize a wide variety of hosts, generally with harmful effects at a minimum. Still, the production of infection in humans can ultimately threaten parasite survival, and certain host defense measures, natural or induced immunity, for example, are necessary for the prevention of long or even short-term debilitation.

Different infectious disease agents utilize a variety of transmission mechanisms. Some agents are carried or transmitted directly from one host to another. In other instances an intermediate *vector* is involved. *Mechanical* vectors that carry disease externally are not essential to the host lifecycle, while the reverse is true of *biological* vectors.[11] Other infectious diseases can be considered non-vectored, because they are transmitted by one creature to another without an intermediate host. In addition, *reservoirs* may take the form of living hosts or particular combinations of nonliving environmental factors. Over time, it is possible to identify some reservoirs as endemic populations. In medical geography, the spatial ingredient is added by the identification of *endemic areas,* and such areas often are further shown to possess common enviromental risk factors. This is true for both vectored and nonvectored infectious diseases.

As explained by Girt, the transmission of such nonvectored diseases as influenza, the common cold, cholera, smallpox, measles, venereal diseases, infectious hepatitis, and others is normally from one human to another.[12] Three major general transmission methods are recognized for nonvectored infectious diseases. The first is simple atmospheric expulsion of agents from one person to

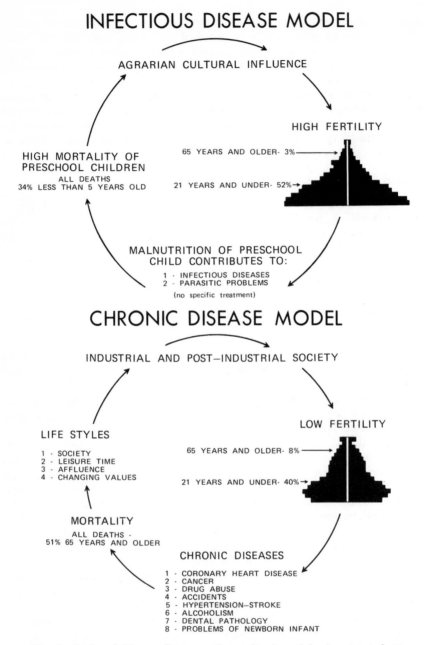

Fig. 4. Cycle of Disease Patterns. Generalized models showing infectious disease conditions in agrarian cultural societies and the relationship between chronic diseases and industrial and post-industrial culture.

another, ultimately into the respiratory tract of the potential victim. Another major route of transmission is indirectly associated with infected fecal matter that has contaminated water or solid materials subsequently handled by susceptibles. A third important method of such transmission is direct bodily contact; the spread of venereal diseases is a well-known example. So-called nonvectored disease agents can, of course, spread via intermediate carriers. Examples include externally contaminated humans, wild and domestic ammmals and birds, insects (particularly the common "house fly"), fish and mollusks. The size and complexity of the living agents causing infection varies tremendously.

Viruses are considered the smallest, and have been until recently the least understood infectious agents.[13] It was not until the 1930s that viruses were isolated and studied to any extent within laboratories. Since World War II, our knowledge of viruses has greatly increased. We know now how important chemical composition is to understanding the nature of viruses. Most viruses have an outer coating and an inner core of nucleoprotein composed of either DNA (*deoxyribe.-acid*) or RNA (*ribo.-acid*). No virus has both DNA and RNA; however, virus-like disease agents (Psittacasosis-Lymphogranulom-Venereum organisms) do possess both. The coatings surrounding the nucleic acid cores are composed of protective protein which also acts as the mechanism for penetration of host cells. New viruses are then produced within the cells and emerge for future transmission. There is now evidence supporting the notion that some of these agents mutate over time, and such change in form appears to be particularly true of the outer coating of influenza viruses.

The *pathogenicity,* or ability of these agents to cause disease in humans differs with the kind of virus and natural or induced immunity. For example such pathogenic viruses as measles and smallpox have a very high successful rate of attack within a nonimmuned population; the same is true of the widespread common cold caused by rhinoviruses. At the other extreme, polioviruses, while variable in pathogenicity, demonstrate a low severity and/or disease-producing attack rate.[14]

Given the virulence, or severity of occurrence, and successful rate of infection manifested by many viruses and other agents, it is not surprising to periodically hear of an epidemic "spreading" from a particular source area to others. Examples in the mid- to late 1970s include cholera and influenza (discussed in more detail within Chapter 5). While these diseases have different agents and means of transmission, they have much in common. Dietz has demonstrated a general model applicable to many of the infectious diseases discussed in this chapter (Fig. 5).[15] Within this context, a *susceptible* (Individual 1) becomes infected at a moment in time. Infection is followed by incubation which, in turn, overlaps between a latent period and one of infection wherein the outward manifestations or symptoms have started to appear. But Individual 2 can be infected by Individual 1 during the infectious period before symptoms have made themselves known. This is not a long period of time in many instances, and the actual lag period or *serial* interval between symptoms of individuals is longer. The overall result is that infections can be spread from person to person before the appearance of symptoms, and with a virulent disease it can be disastrous.

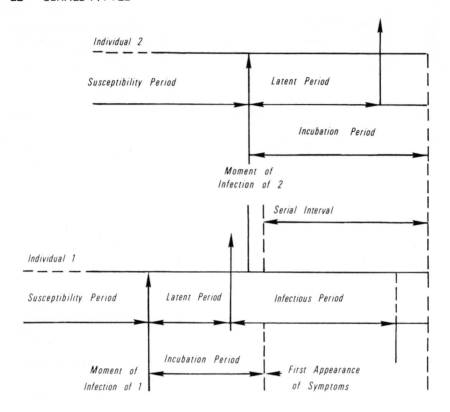

Fig. 5. A model showing the spread of epidemics (after Deitz).

Clearly, not all viral diseases are nonvectored, and many may or may not utilize an intermediate host or reservoir. It is quite common for arthropods to serve as vectors. Viral encephalitis is a good example. Over the past several decades there is increasing evidence that a general group of encephalitis viruses are transmitted by several types of mosquitos and that such intermediate hosts as birds and mammals are involved.[16] Syntheses of studies accomplished in different locations can help explain why, for example, California encephalitis has been considered an "endemic puzzle" in Ohio.[17] Furthermore, such associations are not restricted to viral infections, and Rocky Mountain spotted fever exemplifies a rickettsial disease more common to the Appalachians than the Rockies.

Rickettsiae are a group of disease-producing agents containing enzymes as well as both RNA and DNA. First noted by Howard Ricketts near the turn of this century, rickettsiae are midway between viruses and bacteria in size and form.[18] Four groups of rickettsial diseases including typhus, spotted fever, scrub typhus, and Q-fever, are recognized by epidemiologists. These diseases normally require transmission via a vector, often a tick, with wild and domestic animals acting as intermediate hosts. It is crucial in studies of the geography of these diseases to develop an understanding of the complex interrelationship among agents, vectors, hosts, and environmental risk factors (see discussion of Rocky Mountain spotted fever in Chapter 4 as an example of controversial interpretations.)

Likewise, the environment can be conducive to the spread of diseases caused by *bacteria,* particularly those capable of surviving without the need of a susceptible host.[19] Bacteria are small, one-celled, vegetable-like organisms that multiply by binary fission. While known for a long time, they are somewhat difficult to classify because of a tendency to colonize in a variety of forms. Still, the three main types are spherical (*cocci*), rod-shaped (*bacilli*) and spiral (*spirilla*). As with man, the three elements most essential to the survival of bacteria are soil, water, and air. The medical geography researcher should note that these widespread organisms can be considered ubiquitous and have the potential to contaminate many environmental complexes and diffuse rapidly among human and animal populations.

As a result, bacteria are responsible for a variety of diseases throughout the world. These maladies include cholera, anthrax, plague, tetanus, tuberculosis, and typhoid fever. Bacterial diseases can be either vectored or nonvectored, and this includes the possibility of humans acting as hosts, vectors, and reservoirs. One of the most common mechanical vectors in both developed and developing areas of the world is the fly. Under more primitive and unsanitary conditions the flea and louse are responsible for the proliferation of some bacterial diseases. While such long-known notions as improved sanitation, better personal hygiene and control of water pollution can do much in the way of bacterial disease prevention, aspects of human behavior combine with the ubiquity of these organisms to suggest that bacteria will be "with us always."

Spirochetes represent a threat to the health of humans in several ways. These microorganisms have some traits of bacteria and some similar to protozoa. They cause such diseases as relapsing fever, syphilis, yaws, and a variety of jaundice (Weil's Disease). Modes of conveyance vary because some utilize man as both host and agent (syphilis) while others probably are transmitted by flies (yaws). Still others are carried from one human to another by ticks or lice. In many instances spirochetes are spread via contaminated water or soil.

While more common as causes of disease in developing as opposed to developed nations, yeast and molds are a large and complex group of disease agents. Many are related to bacteria, but are larger and biologically of "higher order." They are often transmitted to man by air-borne contamination or through skin breaks. Many cause a variety of skin diseases. One such agent causes a rare tuberculosis-like lung disease (Blastomycosis) while another soil fungus causes histoplasmosis.[20] Different kinds of localized skin diseases throughout the world are caused by these agents, but more extreme types and cases are found in hot, humid environments.

Protozoa are an even greater health hazard to man.[21] These one-celled animals are responsible for sleeping sickness (Trypanosoma) in Africa and South America, malaria (now apparently resurgent in many tropical areas), intestinal diseases, and many other ailments. Four species of malaria parasites are dependent upon both man and the anopheline mosquito for survival. African sleeping sickness is carried by the tsetse fly with the wild antelope and cattle serving as reservoirs.[22] The South American variety of trypanosomiasis (Chagas' Disease) utilizes lice and other arthropods as vectors with a wide variety of wild and domestic mammals acting as reservoirs. Dysentery is caused by amoeba and is still a serious intestinal problem in many parts of the world, often leading to chronic disease problems.

Helminths (worms), sometimes referred to as metazoa, are parasitic multicelled animals responsible for many serious problems, including widely-studied schistosomiasis, trichinosis, onchocaciasis (river blindness), hookworms, and a variety of tapeworms.[23] There are basically two types of helminth: roundworms (nematodes) and flatworms (trematodes and cestodes). While nematode life cycles vary, a characteristic biological pattern consists of adults inhabiting humans, eggs discharged in feces, free-living larvae, penetration of the vertebrate (a wide range) host by larvae and maturation. The relationship between trichinosis caused by nematodes, and pork consumption is well-known. Trematodes also manifest a complicated lifecycle, and schistosomes (blood flukes) utilizing snails as intermediate hosts continue to present seriously debilitating health problems.

Degenerative and Chronic Diseases

As indicated within Figure 5, industrial and post-industrial societies report a variety of chronic and degenerative diseases leading to mortality. It is becoming more common in such nations to find two main categories of degenerative disease as leading causes of death. While certainly not restricted to the elderly, these classes consisting of "new growths" in the form of carcinomas (cancer) and cardiovascular degeneration are associated with the process of aging. However, certain kinds of degenerative diseases can be indirectly caused by more affluent styles of living in an industrialized society. Additional factors leading to chronic disease include stress, air pollution, diet, and excessive consumption of alcohol. Actually, the leading causes of death, heart disease and cancer, are categorical names for interrelated but somewhat diverse groups of diseases.

Startling increases in the incidence of deaths due to heart disease in the United States and some other western countries are in keeping with the proportion of elderly within those populations. While there are many kinds of heart disease, there are three major types: *arteriosclerotic heart disease* (coronary heart disease), *hypertensive heart disease,* and *rheumatic and infectious heart disease.*[24] Such aspects as differences in the nature of these diseases and methods of reporting mortality and morbidity have combined to indicate a higher incidence of the first two in relation to the third. In the United States alone, more than half of the reported cases diagnosed as cardiovascular-renal have been attributed to arteriosclerosis. The disease is especially dangerous because of the narrowing and blockage of arteries carrying blood to the heart, brain and kidneys. This damming effect can lead to clotting and possibly complete blockage of blood flowing to vital organs. Arteriosclerosis is caused by plaques comprised of fats and eventually calcium which accumulates on the inside walls of arteries. Chances of developing this condition generally increase with age, and there is now some indication that early control measures can be put into effect by lowering cholesterol levels within human blood systems.

While chances of developing arteriosclerosis tend to increase with age, a single diagnosis of this condition is often difficult to identify in an elderly person due to other degenerative processes. The age distinction alone would seem to help explain differences from one place to another by virtue of fairly common patterns of demographic occurrence. Marked differences in death rates do appear among different age cohorts, but there are also strong variations from one geographic location to another. Because of the many kinds of heart disease, there is not always agreement in reporting practices.

For example, a multiplicity of degenerative conditions can lead to mortality, and the heart simply ceases to function. Quite often a form of heart disease is recorded as the cause of death. Accuracy of medical certification of cause of death obviously depends upon the amount of information available to the physician. In some instances, death certificates in the United States simply indicate "heart failure." Still, distinctions can be made in studies in the distribution of arteriosclerotic heart disease on the basis of age, sex, and occupation.[25]

Many researchers contend that hypertension is a leading factor in coronary heart disease as well as hypertensive heart disease. Phibbs explains hypertension essentially as a condition that can produce heart failure due to abnormal blood pressure. Normal blood pressure lies between 120-130 systolic (When heart contracts) and 70-80 diastolic (When heart relaxes). Strain is put on the heart and arteries when pressure increases (220/130), and this can cause a variety of problems including kidney failure, ruptured artery walls, stroke, hemorrhage, and, of course, heart failure. In general, hypertension is also believed to increase with age. It is also found that rates of hypertensive heart disease are somewhat higher in females than in males in industrialized societies.

Stroke (Cerebrovascular Disease, or, Vascular Lesions Affecting the Central Nervous System) is a degenerative ailment closely related to cardiovascular disease.[26] While not always fatal, stroke can be a leading cause of death, particularly in elderly females. There are generally three types of stroke: those due to occlusion by thrombosis or clotting of a diseased vessel; those due to occlusion by a fragment of a clot which becomes dislodged from the heart or vessels of the neck and blocks the cerebral vessels; and rupture of a cerebral vessel due to hypertension or fault of the vessel wall with hemorrhage into the brain. Some studies of patterns of stroke mortality indicate that climate may play an important role.[27] For example, human blood pressures tend to be higher in colder weather, and, in some instances, survival from an initial stroke could lead to complications from infectious diseases such as pneumonia. Conversely, some locations with fairly mild winters also show a fairly high incidence of stroke mortality. In many instances, however, the latter incidence of stroke occurs in retired elderly who have migrated to places with milder winters.

Cancer and other neoplasms also rank high as causes of death in more advanced societies. Actually perhaps many different diseases, cancers have been simply defined as uncontrolled new growths that invade and destroy living tissue.[28] These growths are made up of cancerous cells which differ from normal cells in size, shape, growth rate, and many other apsects. Malignant tumors differ from benign types in growth beyond the original organ. These tumors share the following characteristics: a higher rate of cell growth and multiplication in normal tissue; complete lack of tissue and organ body maintenance; a microscopic appearance that suggests immature rather than mature cells; and the spread in late stages to parts of the body far from the place of origin. Due to the histological implications, cancers have traditionally been considered a collection of diseases other than a single type. Studies of the spatial variability of cancers are somewhat complicated by a wide variety of different occurrence rates recorded by histological *site*. In addition, different rates by site have been attributed to differences in sex, race, place of residence, individual behavior, specific environment, and many other "nonmedical" traits.

Differences by site and sex are probably the two most important ingredients necessary to understanding the spatial variability of cancer. The sex occurrence differences are due to marked differences in male and female reproductive systems, for in women the genital and breast sites combined cause nearly half of all serious cancer problems. When the reproductive systems are excluded, rates by sex are essentially the same. For example, cancer of the digestive system accounts for a great number of newly diagnosed cases in both sexes. On the other hand, one of the leading cancer sites for men is the respiratory system. As already mentioned, chances of acquiring cancers increase with age. The one outstanding exception is, of course, leukemia. A study of the distribution of various kinds of cancers in the Chicago metropolitan area conducted in 1969 and 1970 generally indicates that within an urban area many kinds of cnacers can be traced to the age of the population.[29]

Inherited and Genetic Diseases

While much is known about such genetic disorders as abnormalities of the chromosomes and that some diseases are predominantly genetic, there are also some genetic factors involved in resistance in varying degrees to more common disorders. Still, a substantial number and variety of certain kinds of congenital malformations have been traced to the structure of chromosomes. In some instances, hereditary factors in relation to human disease are manifest in spite of differing environmental conditions. In other instances, environment as well as genetic abnormalities may create problems. Some of these disorders may be caused by something as simple as a change in a single gene. Other inherited abnormalities are biochemical and affect metabolic rates. There are also problems due to harmful recessive genes. Other inherited and genetic problems are caused by differences in blood groupings.

While diseases attributed to a single gene abnormality are rare, one of the most well known is sickle cell anemia.[30] This form of anemia leads to the development of an abnormal form of hemoglobin. Many persons with sickle cell anemia die at an early age. The disease is widely distributed among black groups both in the Americas and Africa. Another possbily genetic disorder which has been studied more widely in the area of medical geography is primary adult lactose intolerance. Simoons has demonstrated a relationship between intolerance to lactic acid and the habits of particular cultures in Africa and Asia in relation to the use of milk.[31]

In spite of some limited research there are many problems related to the geographical analysis of inherited and genetic disorders. One of these problems is the simple collection of information. When certain disorders are widely distributed either throughout the world or among different races (and of low incidence), few geographic patterns can be determined. Even when more is known of certain kinds of inherited diseases, it is still difficult to identify geographic concentrations. Somehow, environment appears to play the role of a "trigger mechanism" for some genetic disorders. As with the approaches to medical geography explained in Chapter 1, we must explore beyond any single scientific determinism if we are to understand more about the geography of inherited health problems.

Disease Classification Systems and the Medical Geographer

Clearly, environment broadly defined must be understood in the search for a better understanding of the major causes of human illness throughout the world. From a natural scientific point of view, the number of possible explanations to human illness represents a vast literature. Research on the natural environmental and human health attracts scholars with a wide variety of interests. It can be scientifically proven that such factors as climate, vegetation, a myriad of tropical insects, and related aspects of environment contribute heavily to the risk of attracting communicable diseases. More subtle aspects of the natural environment, for example, mineral traces, the geological nature of bedrock materials, and specific biological complexes are shown to be having some effect on human health, perhaps leading to long-term chronic ailments. In more developed nations, particular combinations of climatic phenomena and atmospheric pollutants can be explained spatially. The traditional public health approach to human illness is, along with organized medicine, particularly concerned with these natural and man-made disease-producing elements.

It is of equal importance that the study of human disease takes on a social scientific nature. Perhaps the best developed of these concentrations is currently medical sociology, which includes a range of well-defined explanations of illness determinants. The cultural anthropologist certainly plays a role in contributing to our understanding of disease problems, particularly as regards human diet and nutrition. Likewise, the economist has long been concerned with understanding various aspects of demands for health services and the provision of health care. The social psychologist may be concerned with illness behavior to one degree or another with some emphasis at the individual level. The role of the historian in disease studies is well defined, and the literature on the history of medicine and disease-producing phenomena has increased recently.

Since geography is both a natural and social science, a wide variety of approaches to applied medical geography are necessary. When Jacques M. May first put forth the concept of medical geography, his major concentration was in the area of infectious diseases and the natural ecology. Such researchers as Neil McGlashan subsequently expanded May's model and put forth medical geography as "borderline discipline" between geography and medicine. Various commissions and committees have also been established over the past several decades in an attempt to more clearly define and maximize individual efforts in the area of medical geography. For example, when the International Geographical Union Commission on Medical Geography was founded in Lisbon in 1949, primary emphasis was placed on understanding medical ecology. By 1972, the IGU Commission had expanded its goals to also be concerned with understanding differences shown to exist between the distribution of diseases and the availability of health services and facilities. The Association of American Geographers' Committee on Medical Geography, established in 1972, also attempted to define various goals most appropriate to North American needs. Many approaches to understanding spatial aspects of human health problems have thus been defined, some of which are considered traditional and others as emerging trends. In general, research trends leading to applications in medical geography have in fact followed evolutionary conceptual changes within the discipline of geography.

TYPES OF MEASUREMENT

Specific methods of measurement have also evolved with systems of disease classification and trends in medical geography. The International Disease Classification System is now well established. In many countries, hierarchical networks of health-related agencies collect and disseminate morbidity and mortality reports using the IDC system. National states with "universal" or national health care systems are in an advantageous position because methods of reporting are controlled from the onset of patient care by governmental agencies. Still, even within countries with more advanced health care systems, regional variations in reporting exist. Much depends upon the diagnosis of a reporting physician, regardless of whether in the private (the United States, for example), or the public sectors. In addition, hospital-generated health statistics are often more concerned with types of treatment and certain administrative-operational statistics than with disease etiology.

In spite of over a century of international collective efforts in the development of a standard disease classification system, culminating in the more recent impetus of the World Health Organization, not all countries report health information to that body on a regular basis. While there may be many reasons for this, the major ones appear to be: level of economic development, prevailing political systems, and actual cultural variations in perceptions of disease and health. For example, the Soviet Union has a highly developed system of health care delivery based upon a philosophy of preventive medicine. In addition, the Soviet disease classification varies somewhat from the standard WHO nomenclature. The People's Republic of China has never reported causes of death to the

WHO, yet the Chinese have centuries-old methods of diagnosis and treatment. Both of these countries have perceptions of health and disease best labeled "non-Western." Many Third World countries simply lack the resources for adequate health care delivery and have no comprehensive reporting systems. This is particularly true in parts of Latin America and Africa. More recently, in parts of Africa changes in political regimes have resulted in either sporadic reporting or none at all.

These drawbacks by no means prohibit the application of medicogeographic techniques at the international scale, as there are known methods of assessing health hazards in many locations due to our accumulation of knowledge and modern communications. In spite of incomplete annual reporting by all countries, an international system of surveillance exists. The WHO, for example, maintains a regional network of offices whose task it is to cover certain parts of the world (Figure 6). Thus, knowledge of major disease outbreaks can be communicated from most parts of the world, including places not normally cooperating with that international agency at all levels.

In countries with organized systems of reporting, several forms of disease data collection may be utilized. Mortality information in the United States, for example, is normally collected and disseminated in the form of vital statistics. Such data are generated from the local level to state health agencies and ultimately to the National Center for Health Statistics along with other "vital events," e.g., live births, and infant and maternal mortalities. Figure 7 shows how mortality data are handled within the State of Illinois. Major and minor political subdivisions, i.e., either counties or cities, supply information to the State Department of Public Health. The diagnosis must be made by a physician either in private practice or in conjunction with a coroner in the case of death. The information passes through field directors to local registrars and subsequently to the Chief Statistician who in turn is responsible for tabulations.

Morbidity reporting is not handled in the same fashion in the United States. Physicians (public and private), clinics, hospitals, and sometimes various voluntary agencies providing health care are required by law to report specific kinds of communicable diseases to Departments of Public Health. State health agencies in turn send such information to the Center for Disease Control (CDC) in Atlanta, Georgia. The CDC subsequently provides information to the World Health Organization via national channels. This system is not without problems. Not all providers of health care adhere to such reporting, and in many instances it has become "voluntary." Even with reporting, there are many contingencies. Diagnoses may not always be correct because substantial dosages of antibiotics are often administered when some common symptoms of infection are manifested. Often suspected cases of some communicable diseases, or "low-grade" infections are not known positively. Still, reporting of many diseases will increase rapidly in some locations if outbreaks occur. To counterbalance these contingencies, the CDC has established a surveillance network relying upon cooperative sources of information throughout the United States.

Other sources of health data include special studies of designated populations of subgroups sponsored at different governmental levels, e.g., a study of

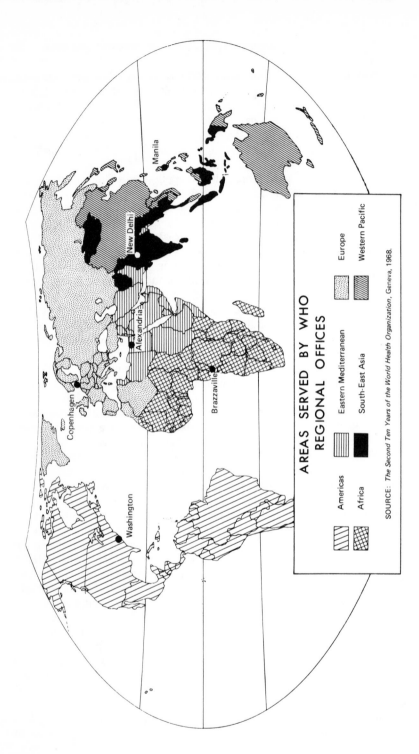

Fig. 6. Areas served and regional offices of the World Health Organization.

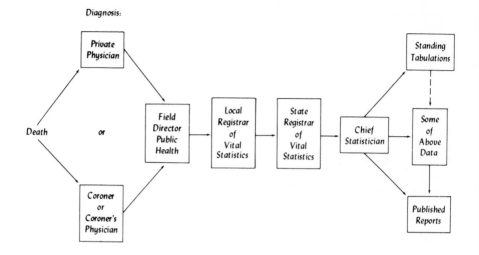

Fig. 7. An example of how mortality data flows through various local and state offices until final release of information.

hypertension of the nonwhite population of South Carolina. Disease frequencies in communities are sometimes estimated on the basis of sample surveys. Also, the Public Health Service reports on the National Health Survey (NHS) on a regular basis, and the National Center for Health Statistics provides the above information as well as additional health data and methodologies for further analysis.

Rates and Ratios

Given the variety of health-related statistics generated in these ways within the U.S. and in similar fashions in some other countries, methods of scaling the information are necessary for comparative purposes, both spatially and temporally.[32] Depending upon the particular purposes of subsequent analysis, especially if data are generated by a sample survey, an important distinction is made between rates and ratios. The term rate is generally applied, with some exceptions, to the scaled results of a calculation which implies the probability of disease occurrence. Usually, a rate is expressed as:

$$\frac{w}{w + x} C,$$

where, w = the frequency of reporting during a specified time period,
    $w + x$ = the total number of persons at risk during the same period, and
    C = some constant expressed in powers of 10 (e.g., 100, 1,000, 10,000, 100,000, etc.)

When rates are calculated, the denominator includes the numerator, and the constant varies in accordance with the numerical size of "w + x" and geographic scale.

Conversely, ratios are calculated in the form:

$$\frac{y}{z} C$$

where "C" is the constant as defined above and "y" and "z" are mutually exclusive. In other words, a ratio of physicians to persons at a particular time in a specified geographic location is calculated in such a manner. An even better example (see Chapter 7) is the ratio of persons per hospital beds utilized for many health planning decision-makers in the United States.

Conventional rates and ratios include many such measures. Those most commonly used are:

1. *Crude Annual Death Rate*

$$\frac{\text{Total Deaths from January 1 to December 31}}{\text{Population at Midyear}} \times C$$

2. *Specific Annual Death Rate*

$$\frac{\text{Deaths in Specific Subgroup from January 1 to December 31}}{\text{Population of Subgroup at Midyear}} \times C$$

3. *Cause of Specific Death Rate*

$$\frac{\text{Deaths Due to Specific Disease During Calendar Year}}{\text{Population at Risk at Midyear}} \times C$$

4. *Infant Mortality Rate*

$$\frac{\text{Number of Deaths 1 Year of Age During One Year}}{\text{Number of Live Births During the Year}} \times 1000$$

5. *Case Fatality Rate*

$$\frac{\text{Number of Deaths from Specific Cause}}{\text{Number of Cases of Specific Cause}} \times 100$$

6. *Incidence Rate*

$$\frac{\text{Number of New Cases Reported During Specified Period of Time}}{\text{Midperiod Population}} \times C$$

7. *Prevalence Rate*

$$\frac{\text{Number of Current Cases During Time Period}}{\text{Population During Same Time Period}} \times C$$

8. *Cause of Death Ratio*

$$\frac{\text{Number of Deaths Due to Specific Cause During Time Period}}{\text{Deaths Due to All Causes During Same Time Period}} \times C$$

9. *Proportional Mortality Ratio*

$$\frac{\text{Number of Deaths of Persons in Specific Age Cohort}}{\text{Deaths in All Other Cohorts}} \times C$$

10. *Physician-to-Population Ratio*

$$\frac{\text{Number of Physicians}}{\text{Remainder of Population}} \times C$$

11. *Ratio of Hospital Beds*

$$\frac{\text{Number of Available Hospital Beds}}{\text{Population}} \times C$$

12. *Weighted Average*

$$\text{E} \frac{\text{Subgroup Populations}}{\text{Total Population}} \times \text{Subgroup Rates}$$

When dealing with age categories and mortality rates, it is often useful to construct age adjusted death rates to be used as indices. Given information pertaining to the number of persons in different age cohorts, the number of deaths by cause for these cohorts and the known average rate for a particular location, the following formulation can be constructed:

13. Age Adjusted Rate $= \dfrac{\text{Actual Deaths}}{\text{Expected Deaths}} \times$ Average Death Rate

where expected deaths are computed by the location rate multiplied by an age structure matrix consisting of age cohorts by geographical subareas.

These and other rates and ratios are used as measures of health status within and among specific populations. They are numerical scales derived in order to assist in quantifying and comparing the constant conflict of living organisms leading to disease and sometimes death. From the spatial analytic point of view, such measures are essential for geographic contributions to the understanding and perhaps future prevention of unnecessary human suffering. In studies of medical geography, broadly defined, such measures are utilized in a variety of analytical frameworks, both inductive and deductive. Essential to these analyses at the "base level" are methods of disease mapping.

NOTES

[1] Folke Henschen. (trans., Joan Tate) *The History of Diseases.* London: Longmans (1966).

[2] Carlo Cipolla. *Public Health and the Medical Profession in the Renaissance.* Cambridge: Cambridge University Press (1976).

[3] Fraser Brockington. *World Health.* London: Churchill Livingstone (1975), pp. 117–131.

[4] Geoffery Keynes. *A Bibliography of Sir William Petty F.R.S. and of Observations on the Bills of Mortality by John Graunt.* Oxford: Clarendon Press (1971).

[5] Johann Peter Frank. (trans., E. Vilin) *A System of Complete Medical Police.* (selections edited by Erna Lesky) Baltimore: Johns Hopkins University Press (1976).

[6] World Health Organization. *The First Ten Years of the World Health Organization.* Geneva (1958), pp. 3–39.

[7] Harry Wain. *A History of Preventive Medicine.* Springfield, Ill.: Charles C. Thomas (1970), pp. 227–263.

[8] Howard C. Hopps. "Geographic Pathology and the Medical Implications of Environmental Geochemistry" in H. L. Cannon and H. C. Hopps (eds.). *Environmental Geochemistry in Health and Disease.* Boulder, Colorado: Geological Society of America (1971), pp. 1–11.

[9] G. E. Alan Dever, et al. *Georgia Disease Patterns of the 1970s.* Atlanta, Georgia: Georgia Department of Human Resources.

[10] Lloyd E. Burton and Hugh H. Smith. *Public Health and Community Medicine.* Baltimore: Williams and Wilkins (1975), p. 112.

[11] C. Gregory Knight. "The Geography of Vectored Diseases" in John M. Hunter (ed.), *The Geography of Health and Disease.* Chapel Hill, North Carolina: Department of Geography (1974), pp. 46–80.

[12] John L. Girt. "The Geography of Non-vectored Infectious Diseases" in John M. Hunter, op. cit., pp. 81–100.

[13] A. J. Rhodes and C. E. Van Rooyen. *Textbook of Virology.* Baltimore: Williams and Wilkins (1968).

[14] Frank Fenner and David O. White. *Medical Virology.* New York: Academic Press (1970), pp. 269–274.

[15] Klaus Dietz. "Epidemics and Rumors: A Survey," *Journal of the Royal Statistical Society,* Vol. 130 (1967).

[16] Max Theiler and W. G. Downs. *The Arthropod-borne Viruses of Vertebrates.* New Haven, Conn.: Yale University Press (1973), pp. 209–262.

[17] R. A. Masterson, H. W. Stegmiller, N. A. Parsons, C. C. Croft, and C. B. Spencer. "California Encephalitis—An Endemic Puzzle in Ohio," *Health Laboratory Science,* Vol. 8 (1971), pp. 89–96.

[18] Frank L. Horsfall and Igor Tamm. *Viral and Rickettsial Infections of Man.* Philadelphia: Lippincott (1965).

[19] Rene J. Dubos and James G. Hirsch (eds.). *Bacterial and Mycotic Infections of Man.* Philadelphia: Lippincott (1965).

[20] Chester W. Emmons, Chapman H. Binford, John P. Utz, and K. J. Kwon-Chung. *Medical Mycology.* Philadelphia: Lea and Febiger (1977), pp. 342–364.

[21] See J. Walter Beck and John E. Davies. *Medical Parasitology.* St. Louis: C. V. Mosby (1976).

[22] For comparisons of African and American trypanosomiasis see Michael S. R. Hutt and Norman E. Wilks, "African Trypanosomiasis" and Zilton A. Andrate, "American Trypanosomiasis" in Raul A. Marcial-Rojas (ed.), *Pathology of Protozoal and Helminthic Diseases.*

[23] Ernest Carroll Faust, Paul Chester Beaver, and Rodney Clifton Jung. *Animal Agents and Vectors of Human Disease.* Philadelphia: Lea and Febiger (1975), pp. 129–335.

[24] The following references were used in formulating this discussion: Brendan Phibbs. *The Human Heart.* St. Louis: C. V. Mosby (1967); Public Health Service. *Cerebrovascular Disease Epidemiology* (1966); Jeremiah Stamler. *The Epidemiology of Hypertension,* New York (1967); Public Health Service, *Genetics and the Epidemiology of Chronic Disease,* Publication No. 1163, Washington, D.C. (1965).

[25] Iwao Moriyama. "Factors in Diagnosis and Classification of Deaths from CVR Diseases," *Public Health Reports,* Vol. 75 (1960), 189–95; Frederick H. Epstein. "The Epidemiology of Coronary Heart Disease," *Journal of Chronic Diseases,* Vol. 18 (1965), 735–74.

[26] The President's Commission on Heart Disease, Cancer and Stroke. *Report to the President: A National Program to Conquer Heart Disease, Cancer and Stroke.* 2 vols. Washington, D.C. (1964), pp. 11–14.

[27] Reuel A. Stallones, "Epidemiology of Cerebrovascular Disease: A Review," *Journal of Chronic Diseases,* Vol. 18 (1965), 859–72.

[28] John C. Bailar, Haitung King, and Marie Joy Mason. *Cancer Rates and Risks,* Public Health Service Publication No. 547. Washington, D.C.: U.S. Department of Health, Education, and Welfare, Public Health Service, National Institutes of Health (1964), p. 4.

[29] Gerald F. Pyle. *Heart Disease, Cancer and Stroke in Chicago.* Chicago: University of Chicago, Department of Geography (1971).

[30] M. S. R. Hutt. "The Geographical Approach in Medical Research," *East African Geographical Review,* No. 5 (1967), 1–8.

[31] Frederick J. Simoons. "Primary Adult Lactose Intolerance and the Milking Habit: A Problem in Biological and Cultural Interrelations: Part I, A Review of Medical Research and Part II, A Culture Historical Hypothesis," *The American Journal of Digestive Diseases,* Vols. 14 and 15 (1969 and 1970).

[32] Most texts on biostatistics explain conventional rates and ratios. For examples, see Byron W. Brown Jr. and Myles Hollander, *Statistics: A Biomedical Introduction,* New York: Wiley (1977); S. James Kilpatrick, *Statistical Principles in Health Care Information,* Baltimore: University Park Press (1977); and Wayne W. Daniel, *Biostatistics: A Foundation for Analysis in the Health Sciences,* New York: Wiley (1974).

Chapter 3

MEANING AND METHOD
IN DISEASE MAPPING

Disease mapping is one of the most meaningful yet controversial aspects of medical geography. To many unschooled in more refined aspects of geographic research, disease mapping is medical geography *per se*. In fact, the term "medical cartography" is used by many nongeographers. To some, the mapping of patterns of disease occurrence is a central theme in medical geography, while to others it is considered certainly an essential ingredient but not necessarily an end result. While there is little doubt that disease mapping is an important part of certain approaches to understanding spatial aspects of human health problems, there are unresolved issues pertaining to not only the importance of mapping in such studies but how particular kinds of information are displayed via maps.

Two of the most important issues, and these are by no means restricted to geography as a discipline, are data measurement and method of display. Yet, these two operations should be interrelated. Many geographers, principally because of training in specific cartographic techniques, are particularly concerned with technical problems encountered in mapping disease distributions. Conversely, writers primarily trained in the areas of medicine and public health are often concerned with the mapping of diseases as central research problems, often with little or no interpretation. Knowledge of etiological agents, primarily in relation to generalized environmental determinants, is used in the development of maps mainly showing risk areas for specific medical problems. To the practicing cartographer questions concerning refinement of cartographic methods are important. Indeed, such fundamentally important procedures as selection of proper projection, depending upon one's purpose, as explained by Robinson and Sale, are not utilized frequently, probably because of lack of knowledge.[1] In addition, whether carefully planned or "intuitively" developed, maps of disease in final form reflect different methods of display. These various cartographic methods show distributions through using primarily points, lines or patterns. One of the most crucial issues in disease mapping though is mathematical scaling of information. Given the same information, different kinds of maps can be constructed showing either subtle nuances or major differences in pattern. When developing maps of disease distributions, medical geographers and those in the medical and health-related professions (sometimes referred to as geographical pathologists) can learn much in the way of mapping single distributions by careful reference to methods developed in the field of biostatistics. Many of these techniques in data handling have been explained by Monkhouse and Wilkinson.[2]

Aspects of cartographic techniques within medical geography have been studied by many. Those schooled in what many consider the "commonwealth" approach have perfected these skills and have offered examples. Andrew Learmonth's review of atlases in medical geography from 1950 to 1970 explains the recent evolution of some of these methods.[3] Learmonth's examples include an exposition of the kind of methods of Rodenwaldt and Jusatz, primarily in the area of worldwide disease ecology as well as the contributions of Jacques M. May in the same vein.[4] Also, a comparison of disease mapping using standardization of age by Howe in the United Kingdom and Murray in the United States is explained by Learmonth.[5] Additional examples include mapping differences among standardized mortality ratios, generalized contours, and positive and negative anomalies as they are mapped utilizing essentially the same data base. In a more recent publication in the *South African Geographical Journal*, McGlashan and Harrington explain a variety of techniques for mapping mortality.[6] The latter examples include maps of absolute numbers, maps of incidence rates, those with discontinuous stochastic variation and techniques of mapping intended to show probabilities based on continuous stochastic variations. Melvyn Howe's contributions to disease mapping methods include the exposition of a variety of ways of displaying the spatial distribution of health problems. Of particular interest is Howe's explanation of problems encountered when mapping particular rates and ratios of different political subdivisions in cities on the basis of population distributions.[7] Howe has put forth methodologies for expressing urban health information in relation to general political subdivisions in such a manner as to present better recovery of disease distributions (this example is discussed later in this chapter).

It is unfortunate that many of these important contributions in the area of disease mapping have not been utilized in a widespread fashion by medical geographers, let alone nongeographers involved in studies of disease distributions. It is still common practice in general medical mapping to scale health-related information in easily understood regular class intervals when, in fact, distributions may be quite skewed. Still, general disease maps produced for popular consumption are more easily understood than those developed through the use of the more sophisticated methods. The researcher is at times simply taking a risk at information loss for the sake of some meaningful form of communicating disease distributions.

Futhermore, the popularization of differential disease distributions is essential to medical geography because of the important nature of such problems and the need to communicate information to a wide audience. Examples of such an approach can be found in the literature on the history of diseases. For example, Ziegler's work, *The Black Death,* is devoted to the spread of plague within medieval Europe with detailed descriptions of the movement of the disease from one area to another.[8] Ackerknecht's approach to the history of disease includes an exposition of past studies followed by discussions of acute communicable diseases, chronic communicable diseases, certain tropical diseases, food poisoning, avitaminosis and several other disorders.[9] Conversely, Cartwright has offered a more general explanation of historical accounts of disease with emphasis on fewer diseases than some writers but more detail on events and conditions either contributing to or resulting from these human health problems.[10] Melvyn Howe's more geographically oriented *Man, Environment and Disease in Britain* is a careful account of the history of disorders in Britain beginning with various reconstructions of prehistoric patterns, evidence of different blood groups, environmental problems during medieval, Tudor and Stewart times, and health problems of the industrial era.[11] Refinements in cartographic techniques and the coalescence of improved measurement systems and mapping are phenomena of the post-World War II period, and still require more widespread acceptance within the medical community in general, if sophisticated disease mapping is to become more popularized.

Regardless of cartographic techniques employed and the intent in the development of different kinds of disease mapping, the purpose of displaying and explaining the information is a prime consideration. Geographical scale, therefore, becomes extremely important. Thus, it is necessary to develop an understanding of the potentials and limitations of employing available mapping methods at different scales. While it cannot be absolutely stated that different analytical techniques are "more appropriate" at different geographical scales, constraints are nonetheless placed upon the medical geographer by the actual information available. The examples offered in this Chapter of disease mapping at different scales are intended to help explain some of these constraints. The researcher proceeding into the application of various methods may want to explore problems encountered in disease mapping. Another goal might be the mapping of disease problems; however, it should be kept in mind that explorations of this nature are also manifestations of many human problems resulting from differential disease distributions.

INTERNATIONAL PERSPECTIVES

As already mentioned, serious cooperative efforts geared toward placing health problems within a worldwide context date to the middle of the nineteenth century. The WHO, functioning as the inheritor of the task of disseminating such information, publishes weekly epidemiological records pertaining to diseases of international concern. Figure 8, containing information about areas of risk for

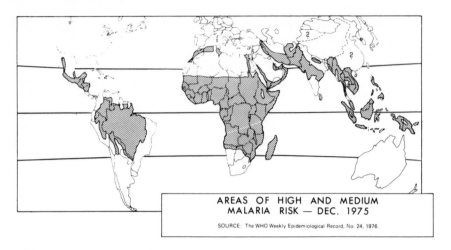

AREAS OF HIGH AND MEDIUM
MALARIA RISK — DEC. 1975

SOURCE: The WHO Weekly Epidemiological Record, No. 24, 1976.

Fig. 8. Areas considered to be of probable malaria risk by the World Health Organization in the mid-1970s.

malaria transmission in December 1975, is a recent example of dissemination of international information. This map was distributed in the United States by the Center for Disease Control in a publication entitled *Health Information for International Travel, 1977.*[12] Travelers to malarious areas are informed through such publications that a prophylaxis is recommended when visiting the shaded places on the map. These risk areas, based essentially on prior knowledge of reporting and known environmental factors contributing to the breeding of specific types of *aedes,* provide generalized information for disease prevention, but because of constraints in map scale offer little information about variations within specific locations. The pattern shown within Figure 8 offers general information about the endemicity of malaria and provides information about a serious malady regularly affecting indigenous populations. The map also suggests that in some places effective controls are yet to be implemented. In general this kind of mapping introduces the concept of disease risk areas from an international point of view.

Risk area mapping can take many forms. Again, on the basis of prior knowledge and environmental factors, Jacques M. May developed many such international maps. Plague, one of the apocalyptic four horsemen, is also a 20th century problem.[13] Jacques May summarized the risk of plague by developing international patterns from 1900 to 1950 (Figure 9). May's primary objective was to show agent–host relationships, but the risk area concept cannot be underestimated. As shown within Figure 9, plague in man during the first half of the 20th century could be found on every major continent. The known relationship between wild rodents (and urban rats) serving as reservoirs of the

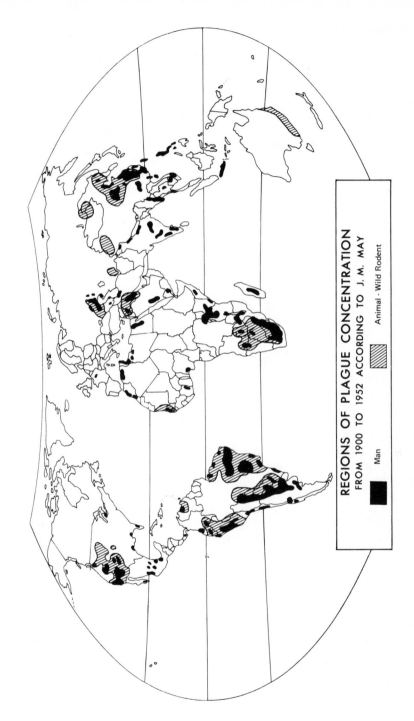

Fig. 9. Concentrations of human and animal plague in the world during the first half of the 20th century.

REGIONS OF PLAGUE CONCENTRATION
FROM 1900 TO 1952 ACCORDING TO J. M. MAY

Man

Animal - Wild Rodent

insect carrying plague to man shows up in this cartographic comparison. By the latter part of the 20th century plague was primarily a serious health problem in less developed parts of the world, with more technologically advanced nations having implemented control measures. United States veterans returning from Vietnam occasionally manifested symptoms of the plague. The pattern of human plague incidence in the Western United States is also of particular interest now. In a recent study, Schiel and Jameson indicated that while plague is certainly not the killer it was during the Middle Ages, there are still portions of the Western United States with geographic distributions of the disease not unlike the pattern shown by May.[14] Such findings indicate the need for continued surveillance and control measures.

Risk area mapping is thus vitally important, and through the accumulation of knowledge over time, information on the risk in attracting fairly widespread diseases can be disseminated. Again, however, such generalized risk area mapping without other kinds of scientific research support does not always supply specific information about human health problems within particular countries. The World Health Organization continues to publish periodic surveillance reports pertaining to morbidity in specific diseases. This information depends on local health data sources to a large degree, even though the regional offices of the WHO continue to function. Changes in the political structure of some nations, particularly those in the Third World, sometimes do not permit the regular dissemination of morbidity information. The United Nations does publish in its annual demographic yearbook mortality data from nations volunteering that information. Since different forms of morbidity can lead to specifically diagnosed mortality, the United Nations information represents a sort of yardstick for use in measuring the international distribution of major illness and how these distributions may change over time.

In an attempt to develop an understanding of such international patterns of disease variation over time, mortality information included in United Nations demographic yearbooks published since World War II can be utilized. For the following examples, leading causes of death obtained from the U.N. demographic yearbooks for four time periods covering different revisions in the International Disease Classification system have been used.[15] These time "slices" include: the fifth revision (1938), 1947 (53 countries reporting); the sixth revision (1948), 1956 (88 countries); the seventh (1955) revision, 1965 (99 countries); and the eighth revision (1965), 1974 (78 countries). Each of these time periods reflects certain changes in the disease classification system. The information for each of these time periods was converted to crude rates.

Four matrices were developed from the information, one for each time, with M leading causes of death by N countries. Table 2 contains the specific mortality categories used. Each matrix was factored using the principal axis method, and after several iterations the best solutions were derived from quartimax rotations.[16] Factor scores were then determined for each of the countries and patterns of common dimensionality in leading cause of death for each time period were plotted (Figure 10). Such a method allows the investigator to

Table 2. Leading Causes of Death for 4 Time Periods Used in the Factoring Processes

1947	1956	1965	1974
1. Typhoid	1. Tuberculosis	1. Tuberculosis	1. Typhoid
2. Tuberculosis	2. Syphilis	2. Syphilis	2. Enteritis
3. Malaria	3. Typhoid	3. Typhoid	3. Tuberculosis
4. Influenza	4. Dysentery	4. Dysentery	4. Whooping cough
5. Smallpox	5. Diphtheria	5. Diphtheria	5. Smallpox
6. Measles	6. Whooping cough	6. Whooping cough	6. Measles
7. Cancer	7. Smallpox	7. Smallpox	7. Cholera
8. Diabetes	8. Measles	8. Measles	8. Malignant neoplasms
9. Alcoholism	9. Malaria	9. Malaria	9. Diabetes
10. Avitaminosis	10. Malignant neoplasms	10. Malignant neoplasms	10. Avitaminosis
11. Meningitis	11. Diabetes	11. Diabetes	11. Anaemias
12. Intracranial lesions	12. Anaemias	12. Anaemias	12. Meningitis
13. Heart diseases	13. Vascular lesions	13. Vascular lesions	13. Rheumatic heart disease
14. Bronchitis	14. Meningitis	14. Meningitis	14. Hypertensive disease
15. Pneumonia	15. Rheumatic heart disease	15. Rheumatic heart disease	15. Ischaemic heart disease
16. Diarrhea	16. Arteriosclerosis	16. Arteriosclerosis	16. Other heart disease
17. Liver disease	17. Other diseases of heart	17. Other diseases of heart	17. Cerebrovascular heart
18. Nephritis	18. Hypertension with heart	18. Hypertension with heart	18. Influenza
19. Whooping cough	19. Hypertension without heart	19. Hypertension without heart	19. Pneumonia
20. Diphtheria	20. Influenza	20. Influenza	20. Bronchitis
21. Syphilis	21. Pneumonia	21. Pneumonia	21. Peptic ulcer
	22. Bronchitis	22. Bronchitis	22. Cirrhosis of liver
	23. Gastritis	23. Gastritis	23. Nephritis
	24. Cirrhosis of liver	24. Cirrhosis of liver	
	25. Nephritis	25. Nephritis	

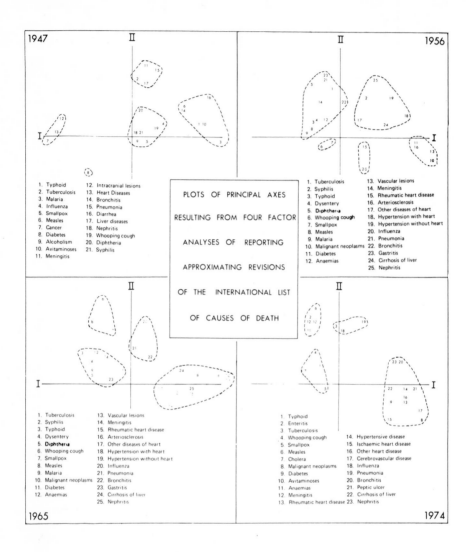

Fig. 10. Four plots of principal axes derived from factor analyses of international mortality information. Each of the years shown within this figure is representative of a different revision of the International List of Causes of Death.

distinguish both different kinds of disease clusterings and spatial variations from one country to another.

In 1947, the fifth revision of the International Disease Classification system (actually developed in 1938) was used in United Nations reporting. Fifty-three countries, the majority of which were more Westernized industrial nations, took part in reporting during that time period. The plot of the first two 1947 dimensions (Figure 10, upper left) shows how heart disease, cancer and stroke mortality clustered in the same factor space, indicating common patterns of reporting. It is of note that during that time period diabetes was fairly isolated from other clusters, perhaps due to certain genetic origins of the problem. Tuberculosis, meningitis, diseases of the liver, and pneumonia formed a separate cluster. Another cluster consisted of measles, malaria, bronchitis, diarrhea, typhoid, and avitaminosis. The latter diseases were quite prevalent in developing nations during the period after World War II. The other major cluster indicated that according to the 1947 reporting, such diseases as influenza, whooping cough, smallpox, alcoholism, nephritis, syphilis, and diphtheria showed common patterns of association.

Clearly, by 1947 diseases particular to developed and developing states showed different spatial distributions. However, during that time period the Soviet Union, China, India, most of Southeast Asia, and a large portion of Africa as well as parts of South America did not report leading causes of death to the United Nations. Figure 11 contains an international comparison of the 1947 mortality data by showing the cartographic effects of plotting negative and positive factor scores against one another for the 53 nations. While the lack of reporting limits the results, it is still possible to depict a more or less continuous scale of mortality classes ranging from chronic and degenerative diseases to infectious and parasitic types. The map supports the postulated disease-economic development association formulated during the latter part of the nineteenth century.

In 1956, 88 countries reported cause of death to the United Nations under the sixth revision of the International Disease Classification system. Results from the two most important dimensions of this factoring procedure are shown within Figure 10 (the Factor I and II plot) and Figure 12. A striking parallel can be drawn between the distributional pattern of factor score combinations shown within Figure 12 and the conclusions reached by Brian Berry in his analysis of levels of international technological development for approximately the same time period.[17] The disease patterns, ranging from higher chronic rates in more developed nations to higher infectious rates in less developed nations, are quite similar to Berry's classification scale (see Figure 13).

Heart disease, cancer and stroke as well as diabetes clustered together in the 1956 data solution. Rheumatic heart disease and influenza formed a separate cluster as did whooping cough and smallpox. Another clustering consisted of malaria, measles, typhoid, dysentery and certain kinds of anemia; the latter diseases occurred particularly in tropical and subtropical nations. Diphtheria, tuberculosis, gastritis, and pneumonia formed a particular cluster within this solution. Several kinds of cause of death formed a loose cluster. These included

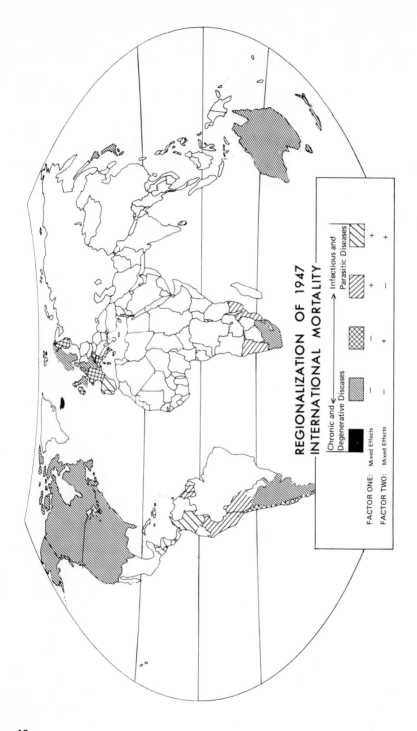

Fig. 11. Patterns of reported mortality in 1947. By combining the first two factors in a scale ranging from chronic and degenerative to infectious and parasitic diseases results.

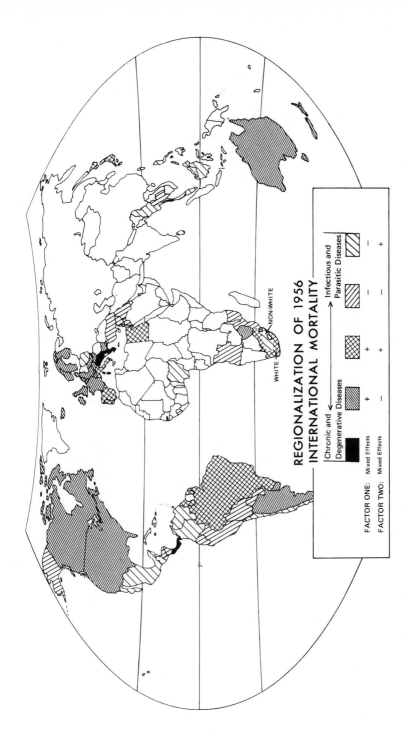

Fig. 12. Regionalization of 1956 international mortality information.

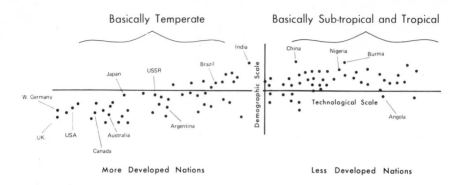

Fig. 13. Berry's classification scheme for countries on the basis of technological and demographic scales.

syphilis, unspecified kinds of heart disease, cirrhosis of the liver, nephritis, and certains kinds of hypertensive heart diseases.

Again, in spite of nonrepresentation from a large portion of the world's population, i.e., the Soviet Union, China, India, and parts of Southeast Asia and Africa, a distinct spatial pattern nonetheless emerged. The pattern shown within Figure 12 offers strong representation from the Western Hemisphere and most of Europe. Thus more developed nations such as the United States, Canada, Great Britain, France, West Germany, Scandinavia, Australia, and Japan showed common patterns of association wherein the degenerative diseases were the most frequently reported causes of death. Conversely, many South American nations as well as those reporting from Africa and Southeast Asia indicated that parasitic and infectious diseases were still more important leading causes of death during that time period.

The results of the factor analysis of the 1965 information under the rubrics of the seventh revision of the International Disease Classification system proved to be the best of the four solutions. Nearly 100 countries were reporting to the United Nations at that time, and refinements in the disease classification system were also reflected in regular mathematical and spatial patterns. Figure 10 shows the results of plotting the first and second factors from that particular solution. Once again, cancer, stroke, major kinds of heart disease, and diabetes clustered. In this instance, however, a larger clustering included hypertensive heart diseases, nephritis, rheumatic heart disease, syphilis, and cirrhosis of the liver. Another clustering consisted of pneumonia, bronchitis, and influenza. The latter grouping is quite meaningful because often influenza and pneumonia are reported together as causes of death. A somewhat loose clustering also consisted of whooping cough, smallpox, and measles, those diseases occurring primarily in developing nations. A related group consisted of typhoid, dysentery, diphtheria, and anemias. When the scores from these factors were combined to produce

Figure 14, the strong argument for levels of economic development and disease distributions continued. Unlike the 1947 and 1956 reporting, rates for India were available in 1965. Not unexpectedly, India was classed with other developing nations. The United States, Canada, Australia, Argentina, and most of Western Europe along with Japan and Israel reported leading causes of death very much in keeping with the public health literature on industrialized nations and disease. Tropical and subtropical nations, particularly those less developed, in turn reported kinds of diseases expected in those locations. A comparison, once again, with Berry's schema shown within Figure 13 helps explain this overall association.

The result utilizing the more recent, or 8th revision of the International Disease Classification system with 78 countries reporting to the United Nations did not prove to be so meaningful as some of the earlier factor analyses. The plot of the first and second factors within Figure 10 shows definite explainable associations. For example, typhoid, cholera, whooping cough, and smallpox, still known to be killers in the 1970s in certain parts of the world, clustered in a similar fashion. The same was true for tuberculosis, influenza, and pneumonia. These kinds of contagious deseases are still prevalent in countries with developing but insufficient health care resources to combat such problems. Another clustering utilizing the 1974 information included enteritis, measles, meningitis, avitaminosis, and certain kinds of anemias. In part, this clustering is explained by nutritional problems as well as general lack of resistance to certain kinds of diseases. A diverse group of degenerative and contagious diseases also cluster with the 1974 information. These included cancer, the various heart diseases, stroke, diabetes, rheumatic heart disease, other kinds of heart disease, nephritis, bronchitis, peptic ulcers, and the kinds of maladies expected in more developed nations. Due to the limited sampling, and in particular the absence of reporting from India once again (along with China, the Soviet Union, large parts of Africa, and some parts of South America) the spatial patterning of these diseases did not prove to be so meaningful when scores from Factors I and II were viewed in conjunction. Thus, while the more or less ten year revisions of the International Disease Classification system continue to be implemented, fewer countries are reporting than had been ten and twenty years ago. Political change, the diminishing role of the United Nations and the lack of acceptance of the International Disease Classification system by many nations has contributed to this problem.

Still, the first factor consisted primarily of chronic and degenerative diseases and the second included an infectious and parasitic grouping. The basic distinction with the 1974 factoring solution was that spatial distributions of scores were somewhat different from the previous time periods due to some of the reasons already mentioned. As a method of compensating for these departures the more simple technique of mapping scores determined for each of the first two factors was used. The results of this operation are contained within Figures 15 and 16.

The standardized factor scores for the 1974 chronic and degenerative factor are contained within Figure 15. The highest concentrations of these diseases are in Europe, while the lowest are in South America and Africa. Figure 16,

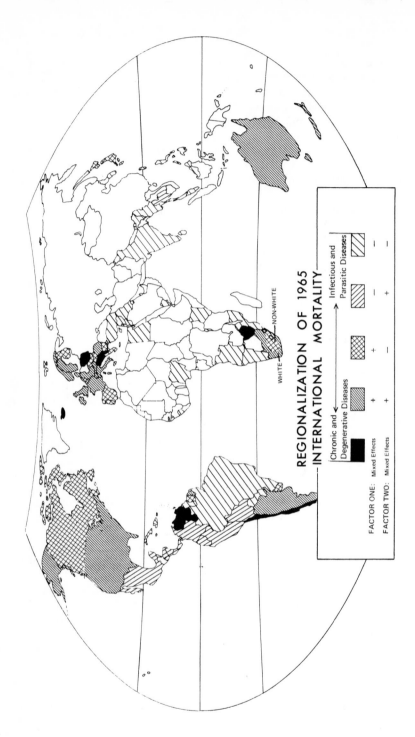

Fig. 14. Regionalization of 1965 international mortality information.

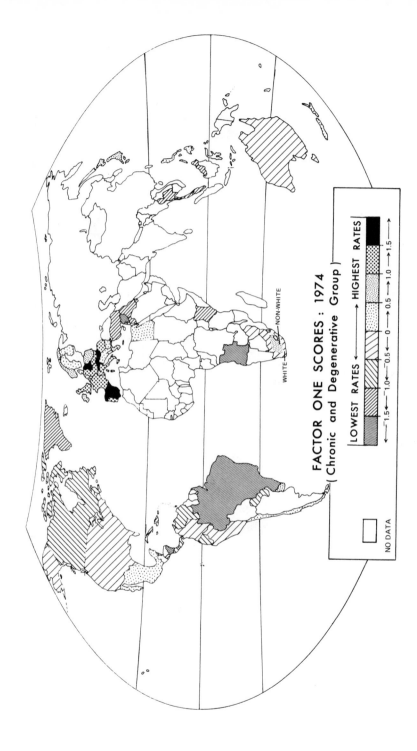

FACTOR ONE SCORES : 1974
(Chronic and Degenerative Group)

|LOWEST RATES ←——→ HIGHEST RATES|

←1.5 ←—1.0 ←—0.5 ←—0 →0.5 →1.0 →1.5→

NON-WHITE

WHITE

NO DATA

Fig. 15. This map is primarily intended to show a range of high to low rates for a group of chronic and degenerative diseases.

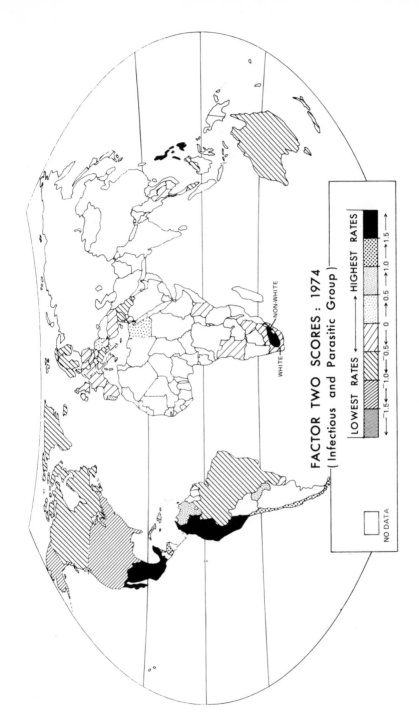

Fig. 16. This map shows the distribution of scores in 1974 for infectious and parasitic diseases combined.

FACTOR TWO SCORES : 1974
(Infectious and Parasitic Group)

LOWEST RATES ← → HIGHEST RATES

← 1.5 ← 1.0 ← 0.5 ← 0 → 0.5 → 1.0 → 1.5 →

NO DATA

WHITE

NON-WHITE

containing scores for the second factor gives some indication of the scaled differences for infectious and parasitic diseases. The most conspicuous features of this map are the high scores for Mexico, Peru, the Philippines, and South Africa's nonwhite population. The remainder of the reporting nations show scores generally expected on the basis of the earlier findings in this discussion.

Perhaps one of the most meaningful findings derived from the 1974 analysis was the position of Western Europe in relation to the rest of the world. Such diseases as heart disease, cancer, and stroke, as well as bronchitis, pneumonia, and influenza are perhaps more serious in Western Europe than ever before. The population of Western Europe is aging. Diets have also changed. A 1976 contribution by Lamprecht and Lamprecht, for example, indicates that heart disease in Europe is on the increase; part of this problem is due to more enriched diets and better standards of living.[18] We thus reach a paradox wherein levels of economic development attain a position where standards of living are actually contributing more to certain kinds of degenerative diseases than was witnessed during the decades immediately following World War II.

The four factor analyses of international mortality reporting give strong indications of the importance of level of economic development, political status and nutrition in the world. The actual mapping method, i.e., using a simple choropleth technique, shows these differences among nations. Given the scales of the maps, it is not possible to account for such factors as population densities and distributions. Other methods developed for disease mapping explained within this Chapter help clarify some of these display problems. If nothing else, this kind of international mapping should serve to caution those drawing major conclusions from international disease reporting. While the statement can be made that there are certain kinds of "temperate" as opposed to "tropical" diseases, the information base at this time is not truly that reliable. Only very general macroscale conclusions can be made. In addition, since the numbers of nations actually reporting has declined in recent times, it is more difficult to actually find out about the status of world health conditions. Still, as explained within Chapter 5, certain kinds of monitoring, particularly for influenza, malaria, and cholera, are carried on by the World Health Organization, and, reporting from point locations, particularly from one close interval time period to the next, certainly provides information about the possibility of pending epidemics. It is unfortunate that even after a century of international efforts such populous nations as the Soviet Union, China, and India are not cooperating in annual cause of death reporting. If major international comparisons are to be made, it is essential that such nations be included in reporting under a common system.

BROAD REGIONAL COMPARISONS

For macroregional disease studies, defined here as either continental in coverage or including groups of countries with general geographic similarities, conclusions are still limited by levels of detailed analysis permitted by geographic scale and cartographic method. As with international studies, it is clearly possible to arrive at general statements about disease and climatic influence and the effects of differential levels of economic development. In addition, implications can be made about human cultures in relation to the natural environment and health problems. Some researchers have even arrived at specific conclusions about human health problems in relation to the distribution of human blood groups. A great deal of caution must be taken, however, before generalities made from studies at this scale can be truly posited as "epidemiological evidence." Placed within a realistic interpretive context, the kinds of information provided at the macroregional scale are not without merit. For example, if diseases are known to be endemic in certain regions of the world, and numbers of cases are diagnosed in regions where they would not normally be expected in some repeated fashion, closer examination on the basis of such geographic evidence is clearly warranted.

Trypanosomiasis is one example of a disease that has been mapped in a broad regional manner. The South and Central American version of this disease, commonly known as a form of "sleeping sickness," is Chagas' Disease.[19] While South American trypanosomiasis is spread by insect vectors utilizing wild and domestic animals as reservoirs, it is different from African sleeping sickness in several ways. In Africa trypanosomiasis has been associated at the broad regional scale with the tsetse fly and cattle raising cultures.[20] Ecological conditions may be somewhat similar in South America, but insect vectors are apparently different. First diagnosed in Brazil in 1909 by Carlos Chagas, there are acute and chronic forms of this disease. The acute form is characterized by fever, swelling of the eyes, enlargement of the liver and spleen and eventual myocardial damage. This condition can lead to eventual heart failure. More chronic cases without heart damage are essentially regarded as intermediate forms.

Emanuel Dias attributed Chagas' Disease in South America from 1909 to 1951 to the presence of several kinds of triatomid bugs.[21] Figure 17 shows the distribution of infected triatomid bugs in South and Central America in relation to human cases. These bugs have a widespread distribution and some kinds are referred to as "bed bugs." There is a general understanding that some of these insects infected with flagellates commonly attack individuals living in rather poor conditions. Infection is apparently more common during night hours and more acute among the youthful population. Given the information provided within Figure 17, it might be assumed that selected parts of Latin America are risk areas for Chagas' Disease. In a recent contribution Kenneth Haddock has reviewed past studies of the distribution of Chagas' Disease in Latin America.[22] Haddock explains how well known the actual disease distributions are in the late 1970s. Rather than attempt to draw cartographic associations on a broad regional basis, he has wisely opted to show where the disease is known and where it is now under investigation (Figure 18). The major risk areas still appear to be eastern Brazil, northern Argentina, and parts of Chile and Argentina.

In his analysis of poliomyelitis prevalence in the world from 1900 to 1949, Jacques May found the disease was concentrated much more in temperate than in tropical and other kinds of latitudinally determined climatic belts.[23] Figure 19, adapted from May's world map, contains a comparison of parts of North America and Europe during the time periods 1900-1919, 1920-39, and 1940-49.

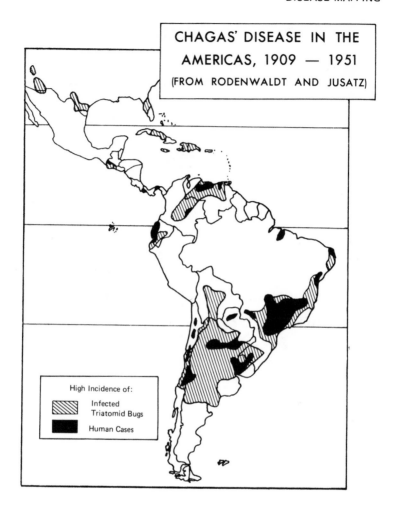

Fig. 17. Chagas' Disease in the Americas during the first part of the twentieth century.

These parts of the world were some of the most severely besieged by the disease during the first half of this century. From 1900 to 1919 European cases were found mostly in Scandinavia and other scattered locations, while in North America the highest rates were in the U.S. Northeast and Upper Midwest. By the 1920s and 30s polio had spread to South-Central Europe and most parts of North America. During the 1940s the disease was most heavily concentrated in the Great Plains area of North America. In Europe, it had spreead to the United

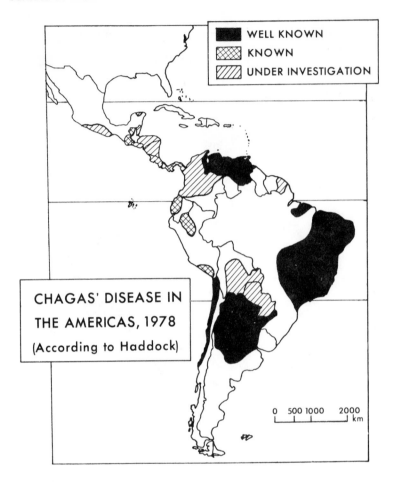

WELL KNOWN
KNOWN
UNDER INVESTIGATION

CHAGAS' DISEASE IN
THE AMERICAS, 1978
(According to Haddock)

0 500 1000 2000 km

Fig. 18. A recent interpretation of Chagas' Disease in the Americas (adapted from Haddock).

Kingdom, and more cases were reported in the North Central European Plains area. Epidemiological research findings leading to the eventual conquest of poliomyelitis placed emphasis on the seasonal nature of the virus causing the disease.

In her studies of seasonality in human mortality, Sakamoto-Momiyama has made some interesting comparisons of regions with similar latitude.[24] Figure 20 shows a comparison of different kinds of seasonal variation patterns in mortality during the 1960s for North America, Europe, and Japan. According to

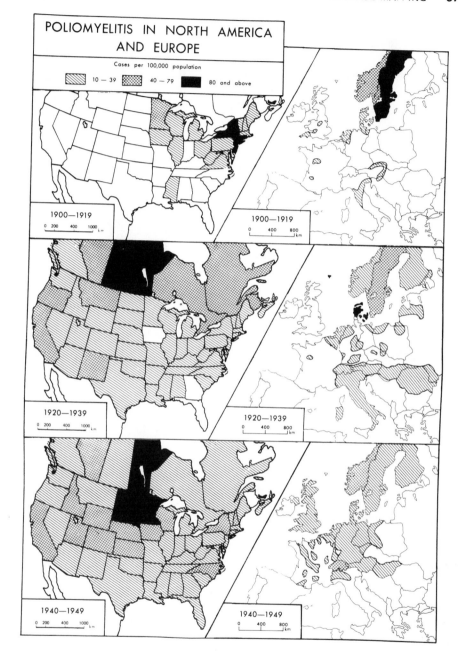

Fig. 19. Polio in North America and Europe during the first half of the twentieth century (adapted from May).

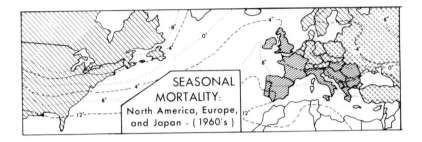

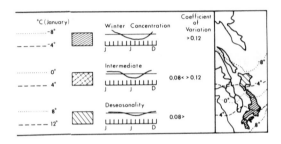

Fig. 20. Sakamoto–Momiyama's explanation of seasonal mortality in North America, Europe and Japan in the 1960s.

Momiyama three distinct classes of mortality "seasonality" could be determined. These consisted of a winter concentration pattern, an intermediate pattern and a pattern of deseasonality. One conclusion was that certain parts of the world with similar average January temperatures may not have the same patterns of seasonality in mortality. For example, the patterns in Japan in the 1960s were similar to the United Kingdom, Spain, France, Poland, and Southern Europe, all countries with different kinds of winters. Conversely, patterns in the United States showed "deseasonality." Given this amount of information, comparisons can be made about the ratio of physicians to population, standards of living and overall quality of medical care within particular countries. However, with little additional information formal statistical testing leading toward valid conclusions cannot be made. This again raises the issue of the severe limitations placed upon the medicogeographic researcher when examining different kinds of health information at the broad regional scale.

DISEASE MAPPING AT THE NATIONAL SCALE

Mapping mortality and morbidity at the national scale usually results in better detail and more accurate spatial distributions for many reasons. Within most countries, systems of reporting death and disease are generally more uniform. In addition, methods of medical education and the delivery of health care are much more standardized within nations. Given a large enough country, there will still be regional variations in reporting procedures, and some problems can result from loss of information accuracy due to irregular, uneven, or nonreporting for some kinds of diseases. Another problem results when units of observation, i.e., states or provinces, are of different sizes and contain different population distributions and densities. In spite of these known shortcomings it is possible to identify distinct clusterings of different kinds of diseases. A major problem in the analysis of disease maps at national scales does arise in the depth of interpretation and association which can be made. It is of interest that there is a substantial increase recently in disease mapping at the national level in the United States; part of this activity is due to the increased capabilities of computer-assisted methods in data handling and automated cartography procedures. For example, the recently published *National Atlas of Cancer in the United States* was developed largely with computer-drawn maps.[25] The Center for Disease Control in Atlanta, Georgia, with its Computer Mapping Section, now provides many more spatial distributions of selected diseases at the national level.[26]

Primary concerns in disease mapping at the national level include understanding units of observation in relation to spatial pattern and how information is handled in terms of descriptive statistics. For example, Figure 21 contains patterns showing differences in reported cases of gonorrhea per 100,000 persons by state during the calendar year 1976. Within this map only three patterns are used showing discrete classes by state. The overall pattern indicates more cases in the Southeastern and Southwestern United States, with moderate rates in the Northeast. Fewer cases showed up in the Northern Mountain and Upper Midwestern parts of the country. Such a map can be somewhat misleading. In this instance, the median, or the measure for which half of the states were below and half above, was 385.4. However, it is impossible for the reader to determine any geographic indication of this central measure. Some conclusions can be drawn from this map pertaining to the prevalence of gonorrhea within the United States, but only on a very general basis.

A more detailed kind of mapping is used for Figure 22, showing reported cases per 1,000 of typhoid fever in the United States in 1976 by state. In this particular instance, percentile rankings are used and class intervals are more detailed. Conversely, it is a low incidence disease and cases are not evenly distributed within states. In this example percentile rankings are very useful statistically, but the map shows that little information can be gained about typhoid fever when entire states are considered as homogeneous units of observation. Such maps have long been criticized by medical geographers seeking more detailed information.

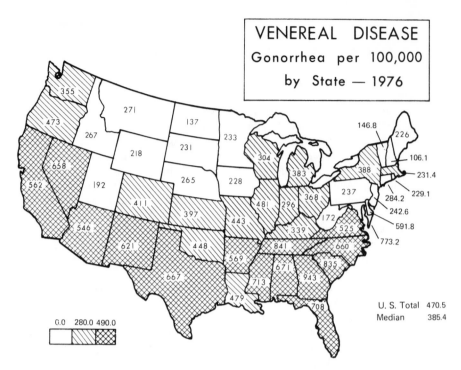

Fig. 21. Gonorrhea reporting by state in 1976.

TYPHOID FEVER—Reported Cases per 100,000 Population by State, 1976

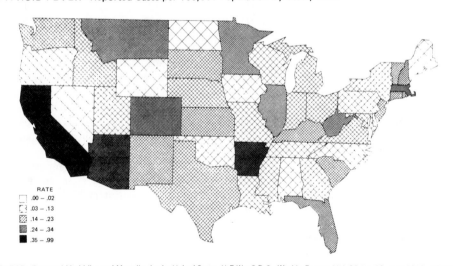

SOURCE: Reported Morbidity and Mortality in the United States, H.E.W.–C.D.C. *Weekly Report,* Vol. 25 No. 53, Aug. 1977, Atlanta.

Fig. 22. Typhoid Fever in the United States in 1976.

TUBERCULOSIS—Reported Average Cases per 100,000 Population by County, United States, 1973–1975

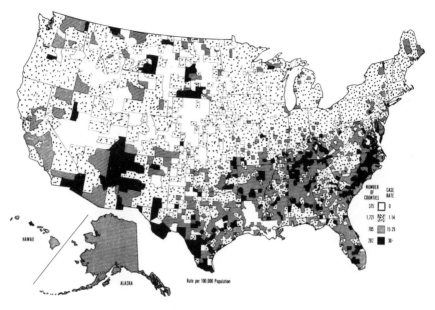

SOURCE: Reported Morbidity and Mortality in the United States,
H.E.W.—C.D.C. *Weekly Report*, Vol. 25 No. 53, Aug. 1977, Atlanta.

Fig. 23. Tuberculosis in the United States, 1973 to 1975.

Some medical geographers contend that the problem of lack of homogeneity within states presents enough problems in disease mapping that counties should be taken as the largest units of observation in such analyses. Malcolm Murray was able to successfully accomplish this in examining mortality in the United States in 1967.[27] A recent example of mapping at the county level is shown within Figure 23, containing reported average cases of tuberculosis per 100,000 population by county in the United States from 1973 to 1975. Definite patterns of localization appear within this map, and the patterns in turn give some indication of the success of tuberculosis control within the United States. For example, the Northeastern United States, the most heavily populated and urbanized part of the country, shows substantially lower rates than certain poverty regions of the country. These latter areas include Western Indian reservations, some of the Southwestern border areas with higher proportions of people of Mexican origin, and poverty pockets in the South.

RUBELLA—Reported Cases by County, 1976

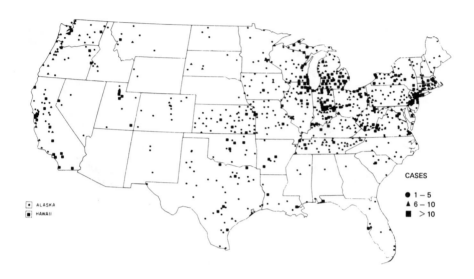

SOURCE: Reported Morbidity and Mortality in the United States, H.E.W.—C.D.C. *Weekly Report,* Vol. 25 No. 53, Aug. 1977, Atlanta.

Fig. 24. A dot-symbol map showing reported Rubella in the United States in 1976.

Another useful technique in mapping at the national level is the employment of different kinds of dot symbols, a time-honored method in cartography. Figure 24 shows actual numbers of reported cases of rubella in the United States in 1976 utilizing three kinds of symbols: dots, triangles, and squares. Although this information is based on county data, a fairly refined pattern of distribution can be shown by this method. Examination of this map shows heavy concentrations of rubella in southern Michigan, the Chicago area, central Indiana, and the entire New York metropolitan area. Other clusterings indicate higher reported numbers of rubella cases in more urbanized parts of the country. Melvyn Howe has refined this techniques to a high degree in mapping mortality in England, Wales, and Scotland.[28] Figure 25 is an example of Howe's work. The actual shape of the study area has been altered to reflect demographic patterns. Howe then uses various symbolization to show standardized mortality rates and makes a distinction between urban and rural areas. In the United Kingdom where such records are extremely accurate, it is possible to develop disease mapping at the national level and obtain reliable patterns of disease distributions, particularly when employing the method developed by Howe.

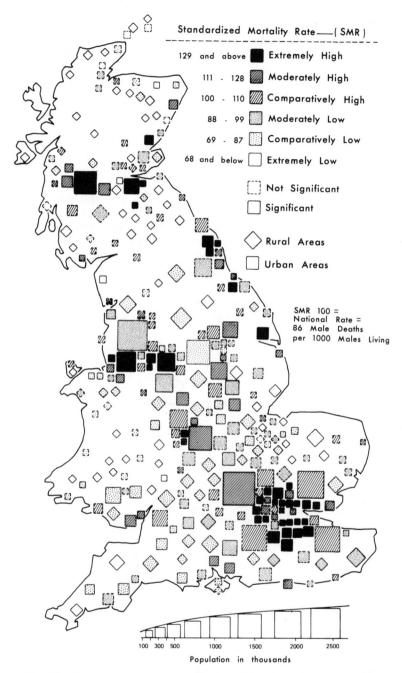

Standardized Mortality Rate ——— (SMR)

129 and above ■ Extremely High
111 - 128 ▨ Moderately High
100 - 110 ▨ Comparatively High
88 - 99 ▨ Moderately Low
69 - 87 ▢ Comparatively Low
68 and below ☐ Extremely Low

⌐ ⌐ Not Significant
☐ Significant

◇ Rural Areas

☐ Urban Areas

SMR 100 =
National Rate =
86 Male Deaths
per 1000 Males Living

100 300 500   1000   1500   2000   2500
Population in thousands

Fig. 25. This map shows one of Melvyn Howe's techniques employed to maximize the amount of information within a map containing standardized mortality rates.

Perhaps one of the most promising methods employed to show the spatial variability of human illness at the national level has been developed by Neil McGlashan utilizing a method put forth by Choynowski earlier.[29] McGlashan relies on the Poisson probability formula:[30]

$$P_n(x) = \lambda^x e^{-\lambda}/x!$$

where x = observed number of cases
  λ = expected cases

The results of the Poisson probability method in disease mapping at the national scale provide useful information in several ways. It is not only possible to show areas of highest and lowest incidences, as McGlashan has done with respiratory cancer in Southeast Africa (Figure 26), it is also possible to statistically test for significance. The medical geography researcher can thus utilize the probabilities determined to explain where reporting has not been due to chance at the .01 and .05 levels for example. One statistical weakness inherent to this method is that more information can be obtained by also viewing levels of significance lower than that conventionally accepted (.05). In other words, meaningful cartographic

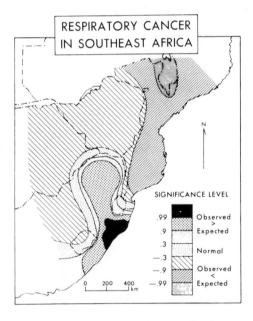

Fig. 26. An example of McGlashan's application of probability mapping.

patterns can be determined by examining significance at the .10 and .15 levels for both high and low significance, for example. This results in better knowledge of disease patterns. There are other problems with this method common to cartography. If a contour or discrete surface method is used, then some detail can be lost in terms of individual clusterings at larger scales. Conversely, if choropleth mapping is utilized, the problem of lack of homogeneity within units of observation remains.

Regardless of the cartographic method employed in mapping mortality and morbidity at the national level, some information is bound to be lost because of the constraints of scale. If decisions are to be made pertaining to national policies and the general allocation or perhaps relocation of health care facilities, then mapping health problems at the national level can be quite useful. As already indicated within this book, the provision of public health services (not to mention private at this time) has not traditionally responded to geographic variations in mortality and morbidity. In some countries, departments and or ministries of health have developed national policies. In others this responsibility is relegated first to states and subsequently to county authorities (U.S., for example).

MAPPING HUMAN ILLNESS WITHIN THE UNITED STATES

As indicated within Figure 7, when information identifying cause of death or reportable morbidity is reported within the United States it emanates from physicians and local health departments and is centralized by state departments of public health. These departments in turn send information to the National Center for Health Statistics, the Center for Disease Control and other related national agencies. The way the information is handled within states varies considerably. Some states have highly sophisticated computerized systems while others are still maintaining manual records. The amount of disease mapping accomplished within states also varies a great deal. In Georgia, the Department of Human Resources has devoted a substantial amount of attention to disease mapping within the state. In a recent publication pertaining to the medical geography of Georgia, Dever has displayed spatial distributions of many kinds of health problems.[31] Included as Figures 27 and 28 are two examples of Dever's useful cartographic techniques. Counties in Georgia are the units of observation for these computer drawn maps. The reporting of acute myocardial infarction ("heart attack") from 1970-1974 has been age and sex adjusted. Furthermore, the class intervals are based on the mean and standard deviations of the distribution. For purposes of widespread general use these measures have been translated into patterns showing average, above and below average rates. The addition of state health planning subareas adds to the utility of the maps for purposes of future planning and present administration of public health programs. A similar cartographic technique has been used with infant mortality.

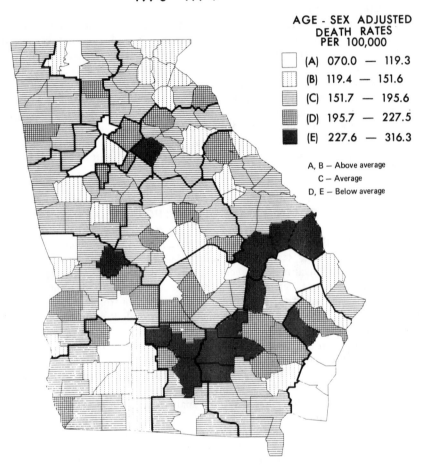

ACUTE MYOCARDIAL INFARCTION
1970—1974

AGE - SEX ADJUSTED
DEATH RATES
PER 100,000

(A) 070.0 — 119.3
(B) 119.4 — 151.6
(C) 151.7 — 195.6
(D) 195.7 — 227.5
(E) 227.6 — 316.3

A, B — Above average
C — Average
D, E — Below average

Fig. 27. Incidence of "heart attacks" in Georgia, 1970 to 1974.

INFANT MORTALITY
1970—1974

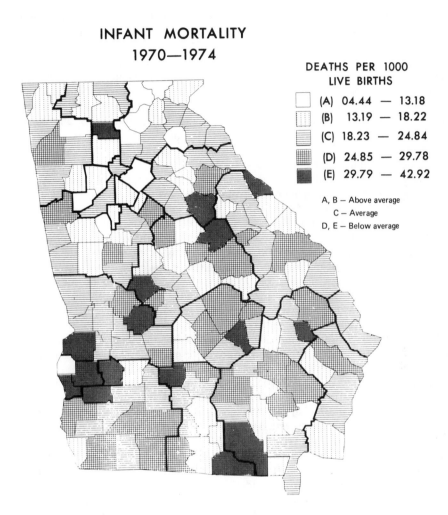

DEATHS PER 1000
LIVE BIRTHS

(A) 04.44 — 13.18
(B) 13.19 — 18.22
(C) 18.23 — 24.84
(D) 24.85 — 29.78
(E) 29.79 — 42.92

A, B — Above average
C — Average
D, E — Below average

Fig. 28. Infant mortality in Georgia from 1970 to 1974.

Given sufficient information it is also possible to develop methods of morbidity prevalence mapping within states. Figure 29 depicts prevalence of gonorrhea within South Carolina from 1968 to 1977 contoured using class intervals identified at quartiles of the distribution.[32] The accompanying graph gives an indication of the problem in relation to the U.S. rate. Also, Richland County (containing Columbia, the state capitol) rates are shown for comparison. South Carolina has had a problem with gonorrhea in recent years to the point where many public health workers consider it epidemic. The state rate (835.3 per 1000 in 1976) was one of the highest in the country. Gonorrhea prevalence within South Carolina is concentrated in more heavily settled parts of the state, as would be expected. Extremely high distributions requiring further explanation include those within the Richland County and Charleston areas and large portions of the south-central and rapidly growing northern parts of the state. It is important when making such simple cartographic comparisons between disease distributions in states and distributions of population that inferences are limited to overall conclusions leading to more in-depth microscale spatial analysis.

One method to approach more detail in disease mapping within a state is to combine contour and choropleth methods in the form of dysametric maps. This method assists in the identification of more specific clusters of some types of diseases. Figure 30 is an example of such mapping, with patterns presented to show California encephalitis reporting in Ohio during below average, higher than average, and average years. An analysis of variance for each of the three years indicated that only for the average year was there significance in comparison with population at risk. However, visual analysis of the three maps simultaneously greatly assisted in the identification of endemic areas of this arthropod-borne encephalitis within the state.[33]

These and other forms of mortality and morbidity mapping at the state level can be extremely useful to health authorities in terms of developing programs for the delivery of health services, as well as disease prevention and control. In terms of medical geography in general, the analysis of disease distributions at the state level are most useful in terms of offering evidence of spatial variations. It is the task of the medical geographer to also communicate that in many instances more refined scales of analysis may be necessary inputs into policy decisions made in health care planning and delivery. Taking the South Carolina gonorrhea map for example, the pattern indicates that the area around Columbia is in the highest quartile for gonorrhea, but it yields little information about distributions within the city. The same is true for the identified endemic areas of encephalitis in Ohio; some appear to be in urbanized areas but others are in sparsely inhabited parts of the state. Having gained such important information about distributions within states, it is essential to develop more geographically detailed cartographic analyses when possible.

MAPPING DISEASE AT THE LOCAL LEVEL

The discussion of Figure 24 suggested concentrations of cases of rubella in urbanized portions of the United States in 1976. Actually, such a pattern was

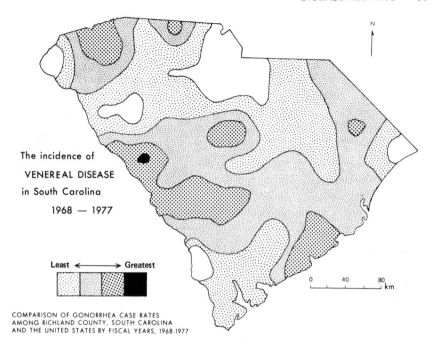

The incidence of
VENEREAL DISEASE
in South Carolina
1968 — 1977

Least ←———→ Greatest

COMPARISON OF GONORRHEA CASE RATES
AMONG RICHLAND COUNTY, SOUTH CAROLINA
AND THE UNITED STATES BY FISCAL YEARS, 1968-1977

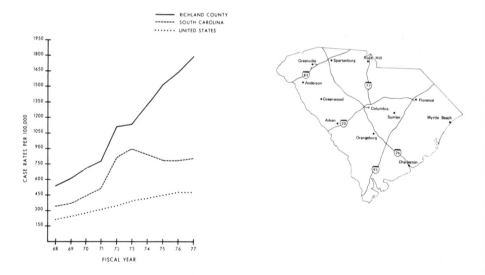

Fig. 29. Venereal disease in South Carolina from 1968 to 1977. Note that it is concentrated in more urbanized parts of the state and the rate for Richland County (containing Columbia, the capitol) is higher than the rates for the United States and the state of South Carolina.

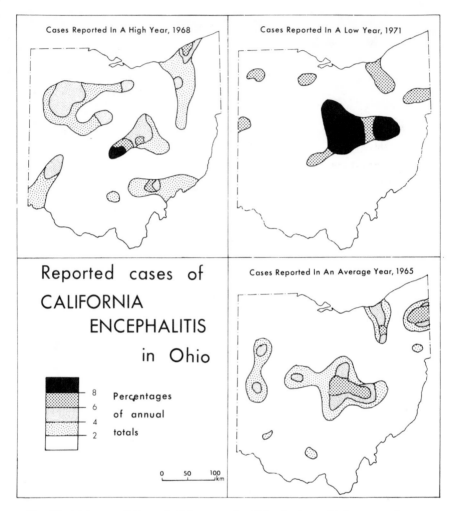

Fig. 30. Clusters of Encephalitis cases in Ohio during a high year, a low year, and an average year.

not exclusive to that year, and it is common for rubella to occur in urban locations. According to Dudgeon (1967), cycles of rubella occur somewhat irregularly in major proportions every 9 to 10 years and in minor or less extensive proportions every 3 to 5 years.[34] In an analysis of rubella in Chicago, it was possible to use temporal disease mapping to identify patterns of occurrence.[35] Cycles of rubella within Chicago community areas were identified from 1958 to 1966 (see Figure 31). During the 1960s a severe rubella epidemic occurred in many major metropolitan areas of the United States. These epidemics were also contributing factors to increases in congenital malformations and the increased incidence of deafness in young children. One result was indicated by increased enrollments in deaf education programs in the Chicago area. The actual cycles of rubella in Chicago were fairly regular throughout the city, but the highest rates were in more densely populated neighborhoods. Given this kind of information, the health-care practitioner can be apprised of parts of metropolitan areas wherein disease prevention programs should be especially emphasized. In the case of rubella, such programs include testing pregnant women. While there are now innoculation procedures, rubella is a particular kind of measles that also occurs later in life and warnings must still be issued when the possibility of outbreaks is known. Knowledge of the medical geography of disease in urban areas, particularly that pertaining to the probability of outbreaks, is a necessary input to prevention and control programs.

It is possible to utilize urban disease mapping for purposes of forecasting. Leading causes of death in Chicago were used to develop planning procedures by estimating the future incidence of cancer and heart disease on the basis of known spatial variations and associations with characteristics of the population.[36] Population density and age cohorts consisting of the population greater than 65 years of age and the population from 46 to 65 were highly correlated with the incidence of cancer in Chicago during the 1960s. Given this information it was possible to develop a calibrated model to project cancer incidence through 1980. Figure 32 is a trend surface of these distributions. Through such a method it became evident that the portions of the metropolitan area requiring attention consisted of the central portions of Chicago as well as the rural periphery. A similar procedure was followed in forecasting heart disease (Figure 33). For both diseases the trend surfaces were developed with particular attention paid to the mean forecasted incidence. Class intervals in standard deviations permitted a measure of spatial dispersion. While such methods are extremely useful in disease mapping because they do show overall patterns within a metropolitan context, use of a general trend surface analysis has been criticized by researchers who contend that not enough detail is shown. In other words, overall patterns can be used for models to predict a generalized incidence; however, the results may not offer sufficient data pertaining to spatial variations within generalized areas of high and low incidence. Melvyn Howe's methods are one alternative (see Figure 25). However, in some instances it is not possible to find clusters of cases without using dot maps.

For many years dot mapping on a major scale was problematical primarily because of the time involved in manually pinpointing particular cases. This problem has been resolved in many parts of the country because of the availability of automated information systems and geographic base files (discussed in detail in Chapter 8). Within the United States, the U.S. Bureau of the Census in conjunction with local agencies has been responsible for the development of nearly 300 geographic base files throughout the country. These files are

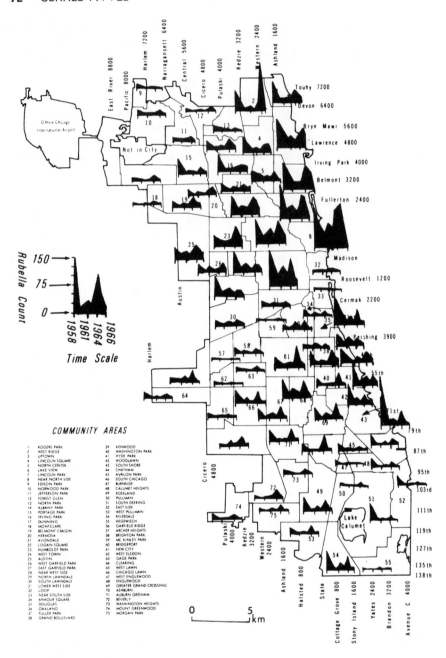

Fig. 31. Temporal distribution of Rubella by community areas in Chicago from 1958 to 1966.

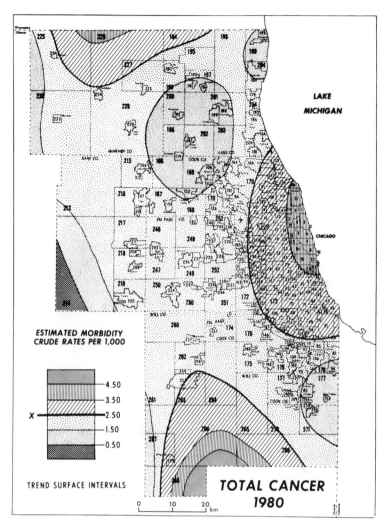

Fig. 32. Forecasted incidence of Cancer in the Chicago metro-politan area to 1980.

essentially dictionaries of information pertaining to ranges of possible street addresses within metropolitan areas. Additional computer systems allow the researcher to take information reported by address, process it through geographic base files and identify locations. These systems have been further augmented by methods of automated mapping using both cathode ray tubes and plotters.

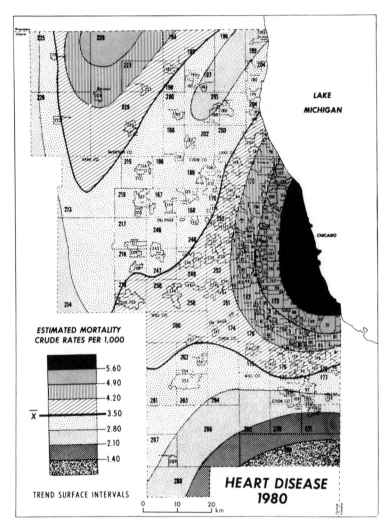

Fig. 33. Forecasted incidence of Heart Disease in the Chicago metropolitan area to 1980.

Figures 34, 35, and 36 are examples of the use of automated data recovery and display systems in urban disease mapping. The state map of gonorrhea in South Carolina offered evidence that metropolitan Columbia was in the highest quartile in terms of reporting within the state. Within the Columbia metropolitan area distributions of voluntary gonorrhea tests for black and white populations for the time period July 1976 to June 1977 are shown within Figures 34 and 35. These distributions were developed by supplying address information from the health department to the Columbia automated geographic base file and utilizing address matching procedures. The resultant patterns were initially computer mapped. One pattern indicates a widespread and perhaps random distribution of white gonorrhea tests. Conversely, clusterings of those black persons tested resulted. Part of this difference is due to black and white residential patterns within the city. At the same time the main clinic within the city giving gonorrhea tests is located in the eastern part of the city where reporting is the highest. This immediately raises the issue of whether reporting is higher because of social conditions in relation to a possible gonorrhea epidemic or because the clinic is located where it is. The information contained within these two maps does not include tests of black and white persons who utilized private physicians.

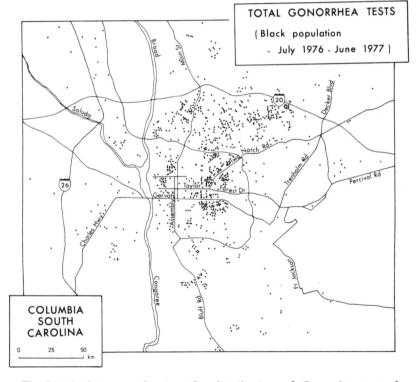

Fig. 34. A dot map showing the distribution of Gonorrhea tests for black persons in Columbia, South Carolina from July 1976 to June 1977.

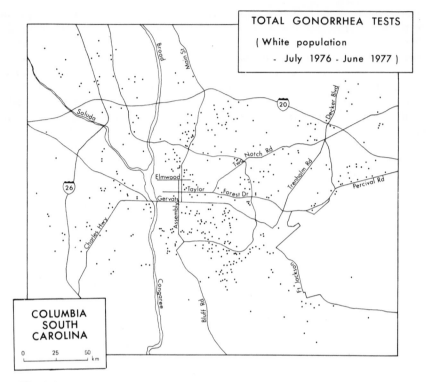

Fig. 35. A dot map showing the distribution of total Gonorrhea tests for white people in Columbia, South Carolina, July 1976 to June 1977.

It is easy enough to arrive at strong statistical correlations between the black population distribution in a metropolitan area and the distribution of gonorrhea cases. Due to the nature of this social disease, geographic evidence is somewhat limited because of the use of nonreporting private physicians by middle and upper income white people for testing and control. While we are able to trace gonorrhea mapping from national to state and hence local level (and use the dot map method considered optimal by many medical geographers), this kind of information is still of limited value in relation to disease control because both public and private health-care facilities are utilized. Furthermore, knowledge of and proximity to the clinic may result in a more relaxed attitude on the part of individuals who know they can be treated.

Utilizing the same gonorrhea data base, it was possible to show the distribution of positive tests within part of the census tract reporting the most cases (coincidentally adjacent to the clinic). Figure 36 shows the results of dot mapping these particular cases for the same one-year time period. Many health services researchers feel that it is only by utilizing this kind of mapping at the block level that any indication of pattern can be obtained. This map indicates more or less random clusters. Knowledge of small area distributions can further lead to directing public education programs on the part of public health officials. Such information, however, is not always available to the medical geographer, and even when available, there is the constant problem of reliability of reporting.

The intent of this chapter has been to demonstrate kinds of mapping methods available to medical geographers at scales ranging from global to the city block. Paradoxically, information obtained at the international scale is the least reliable

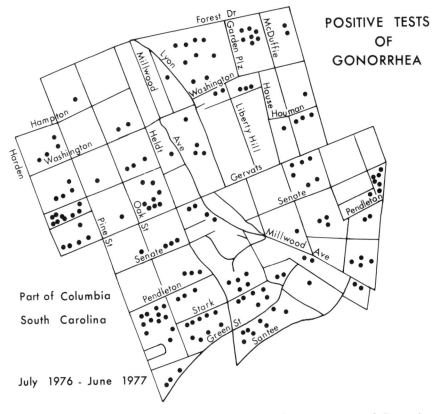

Fig. 36. A dot map showing the distribution of positive tests of Gonorrhea within blocks in a portion of Columbia, South Carolina.

and not always obtainable in the mid-1970s while methods for pinpointing information at the small scale due to geographic base files are most accessible. Only through the improvement of local reporting systems can we ultimately improve the quantity and quality of information at county, state, and national levels. This is indeed a slow process. The medical geographer is limited by available data, and choices must be made in the selection of ways to control for contingencies. While certain kinds of generalized observations and hypothesized "associations" were drawn within this chapter in relation to the explanation of disease patterns, the intent is to primarily explain the implications of disease mapping at various scales. Problems associated with large-scale interpretations unfortunately do not stop with information in the form of dot maps within any form of settlement pattern. As explained within Chapter 2, the scale problem in medical geography ultimately decreases to that of the size of vectors and even parasites contained within vectors. These important aspects of medical geography, generally termed studies in disease ecology, are the subject of the next chapter.

NOTES

[1] Arthur Robinson and Randall Sale. *Elements of Cartography.* 3rd ed. New York: Wiley (1969).

[2] F. J. Monkhouse and H. R. Wilkinson. *Maps and Diagrams: Their Compilation and Construction.* 3rd ed. London: Methuen (1971).

[3] A. T. A. Learmonth. "Atlases in Medical Geography 1950–1970: A Review," in N. D. McGlashan (ed.), *Medical Geography: Techniques and Field Studies.* London: Methuen (1972), pp. 133–152.

[4] See Chapter 1, note 17.

[5] A. T. A. Learmonth, op. cit.

[6] N. D. McGlashan and J. S. Harrington. "Some Techniques for Mapping Mortality," *The South African Geographical Journal,* Vol. 58 (1976), pp. 18–24.

[7] G. Melvyn Howe. "London and Glasgow: A Comparative Study of Mortality Patterns," paper presented at the IGU Commission on Medical Geography, Guelph, Ontario, 1972.

[8] Philip Ziegler. *The Black Death.* New York: The John Day Co. (1969).

[9] Erwin H. Ackerknecht. *History and Geography of the Most Important Diseases.* New York: Hafner (1965).

[10] Frederick F. Cartwright. *Disease and History.* New York: Thomas Y. Crowell (1972).

[11] G. Melvyn Howe. *Man, Environment and Disease in Britain.* New York: Barnes and Noble (1972).

[12] U. S. Department of Health, Education, and Welfare, Public Health Service, Center for Disease Control. *Health Information for International Travel 1977.* Atlanta: Center for Disease Control (1977). (CDC) 77-8280.

[13] See Chapter 1, note 17.

[14] J. B. Schiel and W. C. Jameson. "The Biogeography of Plague in the Western United States," *Proceedings of the Association of American Geographers,* Vol. 5 (1973), pp. 240–245.

[15] Demographic Yearbook. New York: United Nations (1953), (1961), (1974), (1975).

Data		Yearbook
1947	1938 Revision (5th)	1953
1956	1948 and 1955 (6th and 7th)	1961
1965	1948 and 1955 (6th and 7th)	1974
1974	1965 Revision (8th)	1975

[16] Norman H. Nie, C. Hadlai Hull, Jean G. Jenkins, Karin Steinbrenner, and Dale H. Brent. *SPSS: Statistical Package for the Social Sciences.* 2nd ed. New York: McGraw–Hill (1975).

[17] Brian J. L. Berry. "Basic Patterns of Economic Development," in Norton Ginsburg, *Atlas of Economic Development.* Chicago: University of Chicago Press (1961), pp. 110–119.

[18] James L. Lamprecht and Sandra J. Lamprecht. "The Geography of Heart Attack Mortality Rate in the OECD Countries and Its Relationship to Food Consumption," *The Professional Geographer,* Vol. 38 (1976), pp. 178–180.

[19] Kenneth C. Haddock. "Disease and Development in the Tropics: A Review of Chagas' Disease," *Social Science and Medicine (Medical Geography),* forthcoming (1978).

[20] C. Gregory Knight. "The Ecology of African Sleeping Sickness," *Annals* of the Association of American Geographers, Vol. 61 (1971), pp. 23–44.

[21] See Chapter 1, note 15.

[22] Kenneth C. Haddock, op. cit.

[23] See Chapter 1, note 17.

[24] Masako Sakamoto-Momiyama. *Seasonality in Human Mortality: A Medico-Geographical Study.* Tokyo: University of Tokyo Press (1977).

[25] T. J. Mason, F. W. McKay, R. Hoover, W. J. Blot, and J. F. Fraumeni, Jr. *Atlas of Cancer Mortality for U.S. Counties: 1950-1969.* Washington: U.S. Government Printing Office (1975).

[26] Center for Disease Control. *Mortality and Morbidity Weekly Report, Annual Summary 1976.*

[27] Malcolm A. Murray. "The Geography of Death in the United States and the United Kingdom," *Annals* of the Association of American Geographers, Vol. 57 (1967), pp. 301–314.

[28] G. Melvyn Howe. "Some Recent Developments in Disease Mapping," *The Royal Society of Health Journal,* Vol. 90 (1970), pp 16–20.

[29] Mieczyslaw Choynowski. "Maps Based on Probabilities" in Brian J. L. Berry and Duane F. Marble (eds.), *Spatial Analysis: A Reader in Statistical Geography.* Englewood Cliffs: Prentice-Hall (1968), pp. 180–183.

[30] Neil McGlashan. "Uses of the Poisson Probability Model with Human Populations," *Pacific Viewpoint,* Vol. 17 (1976), pp. 167–174.

[31] See Chapter 2, note 9.

[32] Data were supplied by Mr. Logan Merritt (M.P.H.), Administrative Assistant, V. D. Division, South Carolina Department of Health and Environmental Control. Columbia, South Carolina.

[33] Gerald F. Pyle and Robert M. Cook. "Environmental Risk Factors of California Encephalitis in Man," *The Geographical Review,* Vol. 68 (1978), pp. 157–170.

[34] J. A. Dudgeon. "Maternal Rubella and its Effects on the Foetus," *Archives of Diseases in Childhood,* Vol. 42 (1967), pp. 110–124.

[35] Gerald F. Pyle. "Some Aspects of Urban Medical Geography," unpublished Master's thesis, University of Chicago, Department of Geography (1968), pp. 63–83.

[36] See Chapter 2, note 29.

Chapter 4

ELEMENTS OF DISEASE ECOLOGY

The disease ecological approach to studies of the geography of human illness is considered by many to be medical geography *strictu sensu*. Many biological researchers use this approach *as* medical geography, while others with more experience contend that it is, in fact, "geographical pathology" and should be handled separately from general studies in medical geography. In the most general sense disease ecology is considered as interaction of man with his total environment. Environmental associations in disease range from some mundanely obvious explanations to the more subtle. While it is easy to deal in generalities pertaining to climate, terrain, and latitude, this approach appears to work best in a more limited context. Without implying at the onset that many aspects of human culture and behavior in juxtaposition with certain environmental conditions contribute to human illness, two aspects of this approach clearly stand out as the most easy to understand: aspects of disease *hazard* in relation to raw natural conditions and the ecology of *vector-borne* diseases. As explained by Gregory Knight, the disease ecological approach appears to work well in analyses of vector-borne diseases more or less within the context of Jacques May's two, three, and four factor complexes, i.e., the interaction at various stages among causative agents, vectors, intermediate hosts, reservoirs, and man.[1] An understanding of natural environmental conditions is an absolute prerequisite to approaching the ecology of vector-borne diseases in such a manner. The single most important problem facing the researcher preferring a disease ecological approach is the development of the ability to sort out and fully understand distinctions among biological and cultural determinants of human illness.

As stated by A. G. Voronov in his 1977 contribution, "Human ecology thus differs from that of other living beings—both plants and animals—in terms of man's unusually powerful impact upon the environment, which in turn has had an impact on man himself; also in terms of the means that man uses to protect himself against environmental hazards because of the ubiquity of man."[2] Voronov advocates the development of an understanding of man's impact on environmental factors as well as the possibility of man's transformation of the environment in the study of the distribution of diseases. Analogously he explains how it is not easy to distinguish between a healthy and an ailing person. It is also difficult to distinguish between geographical pathology, concerned only with clearly defined nosological forms and the broader concept of geography of diseases. But the impact of environmental factors on human health is not that ambiguous and while many naturally-occurring factors interact, a major goal is to isolate dominant causes of disease in relation to the "landscape." This is accomplished by viewing environment as the indirect cause of disease, or a stimulator.

In the mid-1950s, Jacques May explained the importance of what he termed two orders of contributing factors in medical geography, environmental stimuli and the response of human tissues to these stimuli.[3] He further suggested that three kinds of environmental elements may place human tissues in jeopardy: inorganic, organic, and sociocultural. May intended inorganic stimuli to include such natural environmental aspects as heat, humidity, wind, luminosity, and mineral trace elements in soils and water. The most important of these inorganic stimuli, in the tradition of tropical medicine, May considered to be climate: affecting human tissue directly and indirectly. Direct influences of climate were generally explained by May as the possibility of debilitation due to excessive temperatures, exposure to the sun, and humidity. Within the context of indirect climatic actions, May found a strong association for developing frameworks contributing to the proliferation of disease-causing agents. He explained how temperature, humidity, and drainage variations are favorable for the development of particular parasites carried by arthropods to infect human beings. May also explained the difficulties facing the researcher in drawing strong associations among various human ailments and mineral trace elements in the soil and water.

May considered organic factors to be closely linked to inorganic ones. He suggested that certain kinds of ecological "niches" found within particular microclimatic environments lead to the proliferation of different kinds of diseases in different locations. He also recommended careful consideration of basic plant and animal ecologies usually not considered by physicians taking a more clinical approach. Some of the things explained by May included how some disease-causing agents can and cannot exist outside of other living cells, and how particular kinds of viral agents can be correlated with seasonal change in regular biologic cycles. An understanding of organic stimuli ultimately, according to May, results in placing various kinds of disease problems within a pathogenic context. Related environmental complexes can be considered *geogens*.

While May explained the importance of cultural and social patterns in the provision of a wide range of stimuli in causing human diseases, the strength of his work is not to be found in such studies. Within several volumes during the late 1950s May proceeded within a disease categorical context to explain the geographical ecology of a wide variety of diseases, including cholera, plague, polio, tuberculosis, leprosy, dysentery, and a variety of other human ailments.[4] Advances in medical knowledge since the mid-50s, including the conquest of poliomyelitis, have tended to date some of May's contributions, but there is little doubt that his efforts in the area of natural environmental explanations, particularly when examining vector-borne diseases, have been the strongest English language contribution to understanding what has been termed disease ecology.

In spite of May's important contributions, there remains what might be either a communications lag or perhaps even a barrier between medical geographers and biomedical researchers when examining the distribution of disease. May's encouragements to study total environmental complexes have been ignored by many in the late 1970s. A recent five-volume work on international health problems, with contributions by ten physicians for example, places emphasis on disease hazard in general terms in relation to climate, but differences in illness patterns are somehow justifiably attributed to levels of economic development, and such indices as GNP and infant mortality are used as worldwide health indicators.[5] A major goal for the medical geographer continues to be communication of environmental complexes in relation to disease to biomedical researchers interested in disease distributions.

The Importance of Terrain and Altitude

Differences in altitude imply different kinds of ecological "niches." Terrain influences the transmission of infectious diseases as well as the distributions of certain kinds of degenerative diseases. One such example is the ecology of Burkitt's Lymphoma. This disease, now best understood in Africa, is manifested by tumorous masses commonly in the region of the jaw but also found in other histological sites.[6] The first definitive description of this malady was offered by Burkitt in 1958 after more than a half century of research. The disease has particularly high incidence in tropical Africa and New Guinea, but cases have more recently been found in other parts of the world including childhood lymphomas in the United States. Not all tumors are malignant, and many can be removed through modern methods of treatment. In an examination of the geographical distribution of this disease, Dennis Burkitt explained the endemnicity in terms of a "lymphoma belt" straddling the Equator in Africa (Figure 37). Particularly detailed studies were accomplished in East Africa where it was contended that the incidence of the disease decreased with higher altitudes. According to A. J. Haddow, rainfall and altitude were important ingredients to understanding incidence of the disease or lack thereof in Africa.[7] While the disease is widely distributed in tropical rainforests in West and Central Africa, there is an apparent altitude barrier at approximately 3,000 feet in East Africa. However, a more recent study by McGlashan in 1969 placed the elevation

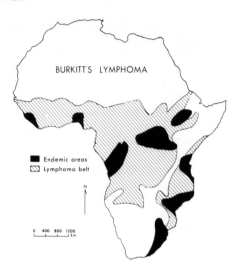

Fig. 37. Generalized Lymphoma Belt
identified in Africa with endemic areas.

level at from 1,500 to 2,000 feet higher than that originally suggested by Burkitt.[8]

In addition to African studies, Haddow examined the distribution of Burkitt's Lymphoma in New Guinea. After such a comparative analysis, Haddow put forth the notion that not only climate but also particular insect vectors may somehow be associated with the distribution of the disease and that there may be an infective agent involved. Haddow contended that in areas where there are strong seasonal differences in rainfall, a break would occur in the transmission of viruses carried by different kinds of *Anopheles*. He added support to his argument by comparing the distribution of Burkitt's Lymphoma to differences in environmental factors contributing to the presence of vectors with African trypanosomiasis (Tsetse flies). Some *Anopheles* eradication programs apparently have not seriously lowered the incidence of the lymphoma. This is explained by Haddow in attempting to equate Burkitt's Lymphoma with particular vectors as due to the possibility that the disease is spread by multiple vectors. Such explanation takes into account different kinds of mosquitoes found in many parts of the world. In general, Haddow suggests the absence of tumors in some parts of Africa is because of the lack of suitable environmental conditions for the proliferation of insect vectors.

In another contribution pertaining to disease ecology and altitude, Robert Roundy has explained Ethiopian disease hazards in relation to altitudinal mobility.[9] Ethiopia is a country with substantial topographic variations. As explained by Roundy, while altitude has a constraining effect on the endemicity of different kinds of diseases, movements of human populations for various reasons from one altitude to another offers exposure to many diseases. Figure 38 assists in explaining these disease hazards. Roundy classified human population movements by reason as well as intensity in his research. Endemic foci considered included schistosomiasis, malaria, yellow fever, and yaws. Such human activities as farming and herding, for example, carried out on a very regular basis, leads to exposure to schistosomiasis and malaria. Certain social activities might contribute to disease hazard but on a less regular basis. Roundy's findings in Ethiopia add support to the studies of Yelizarov on the medical geography of that country.[10] Figure 39, for example, shows Yelizarov's interpretation of schistosomiasis endemicity within Ethiopia. Given the deeply disected nature of the terrain, the prevalence of schistosomiasis in lower altitude river valleys stands out quite sharply.

One specific human ailment that can be explained by natural geographic phenomena, particularly terrain in relation to the geochemical environment, is goitre. It is now well established that iodine deficiency plays a major role in the probability of humans and some animals developing a goitre. Given worldwide control measures and programs geared toward the dissemination of iodized salt, the worldwide incidence of goitre has been substantially reduced. Still, there are many parts of the world wherein goitre remains endemic, and it is through geographical analyses of these areas that we can develop an even greater understanding of the disease. Several recent studies of a medical geographic nature have examined endemic goitre in different parts of the world. In 1975, Ishankulov, Aydarkhanov, and Zel'tser explained natural cause and effect relationships and goitre in Southeastern Kazakhstan.[11] Scheil and Wepfer published a survey study of goitre in the United States in 1976,[12] and more recently Akhtar has developed an analysis of goitre in the Kumaon region of India.[13] Including iodine deficiency, there are four theories pertaining to the incidence of goitre. The other three include the excessive presence of minerals in water (calcium and fluoride), the possibility of attracting goitre through ingestion of food and water exposed to the *Brassicia* species (cruciferous plants) and a yet unexplored theory suggesting that some forms of goitre may be infectious. Soviet medical geographers examining endemic goitre in Southeastern Kazakhstan attributed the disease to a complex of many environmental phenomena. These included, of course, iodine deficiency, carbonate accumulation, excessive leaching, poor drainage, the seasonality of rainfall and other forms of moisture, fluvial action, and the presence of glaciated land forms. It is of particular interest that the three areas studied by the American, Soviet, and Indian medical geographers are parts of the world that experienced different degrees of Pleistocene glaciation (Figure 40). The effects of glaciation include thinner soils and the removal of many kinds of chemicals. Glaciation in conjunction with particular kinds of bedrock, especially calcareous in nature, may indeed explain much about the endemicity of untreated goitre in the world. While iodine prophylaxis is known to be the answer, the aspect of identification of trace elements in local water supplies represents a challenge to medical geographers in the study of goitre as well as other forms of disease.

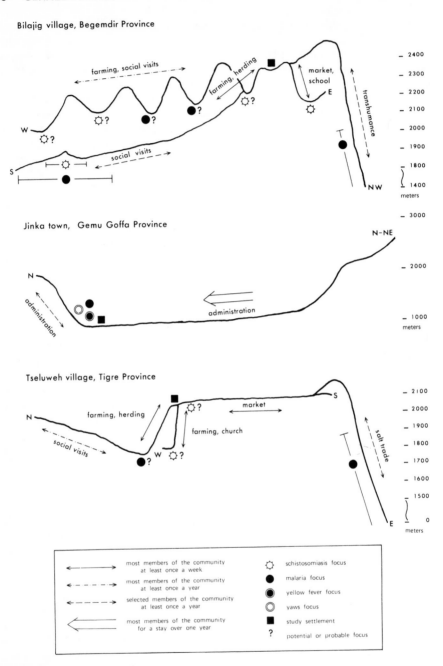

Fig. 38. Robert Roundy's explanation of disease risk in relation to altitude in parts of Ethiopia.

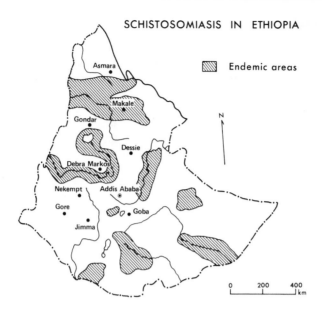

Fig. 39. Endemic areas of Schistosomiasis in Ethiopia.

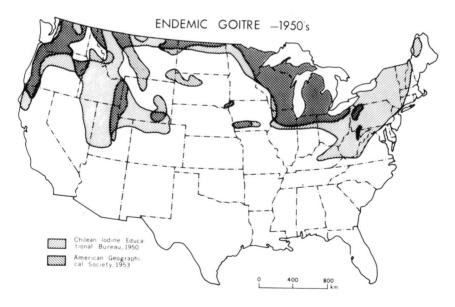

Fig. 40. Endemic Goitre in the first part of the twentieth century in the United States (after Schiel and Wepfer).

Geochemical Explanations

A substantial literature exists pertaining to the geochemical environment and human health and disease. In a 1972 publication, Robert Mitchell placed the total trace element approach into context by explaining general relationships among such natural features as bedrock type, water, pollution, animal food, soil additives, plants, and man's ingestion of food and water.[14] Human ingestion of food and water varies tremendously from one society to another. In highly localized agrarian cultures where most water supplies are within walking distance and foods consumed by inhabitants are grown within garden plots, more meaningful associations can be drawn. However, there are substantially fewer detailed investigations carried on in these areas. Most studies appear to be related to more industrialized nations. The most precise findings have resulted from autopsies of humans carried on in Canada, London, and Glasgow.

These kinds of studies in medical geography are essentially of two types: those pertaining to trace elements in soils cycled through plant and animal food to humans and the chemical nature of water supplies. Mitchell has explained the process whereby certain trace elements can be transferred from soils to plant roots and ultimately diffused into human systems. Following this logic in a 1967 publication Warren, DeLavault, and Cross tested the possible relationship between geology and certain disease patterns.[15] These associations include multiple sclerosis in Norway, Sweden, Denmark, many parts of the British Isles, and Switzerland. They paid particular attention to copper, zinc, lead, and molybdenum in soils. In a more recent study Harry Warren examined the same metals and compared British and Canadian examples in relation to common garden vegetables such as lettuce, cabbage, potatoes, beans, carrots, and beets.[16] While these metals are known to have a variety of deleterious effects on humans sampling can be difficult in such studies because soils vary so much within locations. In two studies edited by Cannon and Hopps a variety of trace elements were examined in relation to the incidence of such degenerative diseases as cancer, heart disease, and stroke.[17] Armstrong has criticized this approach to some extent, particularly on the basis of generalized mapping and the inadequacy in statistical testing.[18]

One aspect of this approach clearly stands out. The presence of different trace elements, particularly in water, is known to lead to certain kinds of disease. As pointed out by The National Academy of Science in 1976, there has been a resurgence of scientific attention in the area of water hardness (or softness) and cardiovascular disease.[19] Several trace elements have been examined. For example, magnesium is known to be one of the major constituents of hardness of water, and this mineral was not associated with mortality rates in England and Wales. At issue is just exactly how hard and soft water are defined in relation to magnesium. Additional elements to be considered include lead and cadmium, copper and zinc, and fluoride. The largest single problem with researching such studies is that we are relying heavily on the indirect effects of environment. In a recent review of this literature by Corbett, he arrived at the following conclusions:[20]

1. No clear relation has been established between terrain conditions and natural water sources in relation to trace elements.
2. Rainfall, particularly in semi-arid areas, causes the accumulation of particular kinds of salts.
3. Many major stream types contain water of the calcium-bicarbonate variety, and the degree of bedrock solubility in relation to terrain and time contribute to the number of trace elements.
4. Ground water is more apt to contain trace elements from local rock materials.
5. Areas near oceans tend to contain more salt than local water due to sodium chloride associations.
6. The hydrologic cycle must be taken into consideration when examining trace elements in water; this includes rainfall, weathering, and evaporation.
7. In general, a review of most of the waters in the United States reveals high concentrations of calcium, magnesium, carbonates, and bicarbonates.

Clearly, many aspects of the geochemical environment must be better understood if such studies are to be pursued in greater detail. Investigations ideally would include teams of experts incorporating those with skills in medical geography. There are also important questions about data acquisition, sampling, and testing for significant relationships. While there is little doubt that trace elements can seriously affect human health, no widespread policy actions can be effective without a substantial amount of geographic information.

Pragmatic Applications in Medical Geography: The Soviet Thrust

For nearly two decades Soviet geographers have been working with physicians devoting attention to what they term medical geographic studies of Russian territories. In a 1964 methodological contribution by Shoshin, the sanctions to pragmatically-oriented studies were given in the form of a mandate by the Central Committee of the Communist Party and the Council of Ministers of the U.S.S.R. in January 1960.[21] Actually, Shoshin traces Soviet interests through most of this century with particular emphasis on the late 1940s as a formative period. While all centering about natural environmental aspects of human illness, Soviet studies take several forms. For example, both Shoshin and Ignat'yev formalized methodological statements pertaining to what should be studied in the area of medical geography in the mid-1960s.[22] According to Shoshin, medical geographic research should be designed to study the effect of the geographical environment on human health problems. Methods of investigation should include mapping of particular kinds of disease. Kinds of information should also, according to Shoshin, include information about geomorphology, population geography, climatology, soil science, geobotany, and zoogeography. These aspects should be interrelated to the science of disease etiology. Shoshin states the following trends are being utilized in Soviet medical geography:

1. The evaluation of individual components of natural conditions.

2. The study of landscape regions, i.e., natural complexes, in relation to the distribution of diseases.
3. Geographical studies of individual diseases, including spatial distributions and the identification of endemic areas.
4. Evaluating the complex natural and social-economic conditions of individual parts of the country to the end that effective public health programs can be operationalized.

One recent Soviet thrust in medical geography is intended to incorporate information derived from the basis of environmental studies as inputs to planning for the development of new territories within the country. In one such statement Ignat'yev suggested that certain geographic information could be used to simulate or forecast disease problems in new development areas.[23] Based on experiences in Siberia and the Soviet Far East, Ignat'yev stressed the importance of geographic environment in relation to new area development. At that time Ignat'yev espoused the theory that medical geographic forecasting should be an integral part of any new development plans in the Soviet Union. By forecasting, Ignat'yev meant the development of disease distribution maps in conjunction with influencing components of the natural environment. This step would be followed by two additional ones geared toward the formulation of regional development plans and new construction projects on the basis of disease risks. In essence, the Soviet philosophy of transformation of environment and the possible consequences on humans is reflected in the methodological statements of both Shoshin and Ignat'yev.

Following that logic, Khlebovich, Chudnova, and Soboleva examined the expanding oil industry in the Middle Ob Valley of Western Siberia in relation to health problems resulting from the opening of new areas of natural resources in that part of the country.[24] The resultant major influx of population caused a need for understanding potential health problems in that diverse environment. The natural environment of the Ob region was therefore studied along with information pertaining to the overall incidence of disease. In order to accomplish this the authors were concerned about temperatures, drainage, and various kinds of insects in the area. A nosologic profile of oil and lumber workers in that particular area indicated that one major problem consisted of overexposure to extreme temperatures. Additional problems consisted of chronic ailments of the digestive tract, respiratory problems, and some circulatory problems. These authors advocated a comparative study of humans native to the area in relation to inmigrants in attempting to explain the effects of natural environment and human health.

In a more recent study of the Ust'-Ilimsk industrial area Soboleva offered similar natural environmental information, particularly pertaining to climate as a necessary ingredient in the planning process.[25] Since it was assumed in 1974 that the construction of a hydroelectric station in that part of the taiga would stimulate rapid growth of industry and influxes in population, an analysis of the probable effects of harsh climate on humans was undertaken by Soboleva. In addition, aspects of the geochemical environment, i.e., known shortages in iodine and fluorine were examined. Again, some endemism of goitre was identified in the natural inhabitants of that area.

Soviet studies in medical geography developed prior to the methodological statements of Shoshin and Ignat'yev were much less pragmatically oriented but nonetheless concerned with providing information about natural habitats. For example, in 1962, Byakov examined the effect of mountain climates, solar radiation, soil, water, and plant life on human organisms. Byakov paid particular attention to certain kinds of environmental conditions in low, middle, and high altitude mountains and highlands and their effects on humans.[26] According to Byakov, the character of mountain relief determines to some extent climate, which ultimately has an effect on human settlement. Byakov was concerned with, among other things, the effects of hypoxemia (oxygen deficiency) and human performance at higher altitudes. In addition, some analysis of differential cardiovascular activity was examined in relation to altitude. Byakov indicated certain changes in glandular secretions as well as general metabolistic changes in humans with varying altitudes. He was also concerned with temperature variations in mountain landscapes and the presence of particular kinds of bacteria. Vegetation was studied in relation to the geochemistry of soils in various mountain habitats. Various kinds of arthropods were also examined in relation to their potential as disease vectors. In a similar kind of study, G. T. Ivanov provided a compendium of data in 1962 about medical geographic conditions in the northern parts of the European RSFSR.[27] This study included an analysis of water, soil, and climate in the northern parts of the Soviet Union. Some attention was paid to human circulatory problems in extreme cold conditions as well. The earlier studies by Ivanov and Byakov were much more oriented toward biogeographic aspects of specific environments in the Soviet Union, and this kind of information was ultimately used in the more recent planning-oriented pragmatic studies.

In spite of years of attempting to develop a full understanding of etiological complexes in relation to various aspects of the natural environment, it has become increasingly clear that aspects of climate cannot be separated from any of these approaches. The Soviet examples demonstrate this to an extreme. In order to truly understand biogeographic complexes, particularly those in a natural state, leading to human disease problems there is little doubt that climatic considerations must be taken into consideration. The most pressing issue in relation to climate and medical geography is degree of emphasis. Without some degree of caution, we might end up replicating some of the general inventories produced during the 1930s and 1940s. Still, the best understood disease ecological associations place heavy emphasis on climate.

Examples of the Influence of Climate

Malaria is a disease about which we have known a great deal for nearly a century, but it still poses a problem to man in terms of morbidity, mortality, and long-term debilitation. The geogrpahic parameters of malaria have been thoroughly studied and include such broad delimiting factors as rainfall, humidity, altitude, latitude, and temperatures: all amenable to the breeding of more than 80 different kinds of *Anopheles.* Reference back to Figure 8 gives some general indication of malaria risk internationally. Jacques May termed malaria a three-factor disease, i.e., one including agent, host, and vector. Major contributions to the understanding of the ecology of malaria were made at the end of the 19th and beginning of the 20th centuries.[28] There are four known agents of the malaria parasite (class *Sporazoa* and genus *Plasmodium*). The four main species affecting man include *Plasmodium malarie* discovered in the early 1880s, *Plasmodium vivax* identified in 1890, *Plasmodium falciparum* (1897), and *Plasmodium ovale* (1922). There is a definite malaria cycle which can be attributed to the breeding cycles of various kinds of anopheles, and subsequently the four major parasites. The lives of the parasites can be divided into asexual and sexual phases. The sexual phase (sporogony) takes place in the mosquito. The female anophalene ingests blood meal from infected vertebrate hosts. Exflagellation takes place following ingestion wherein male cells attach themselves and seek out female cells. Sexual fusion occurs and a fertilized form of the parasite (zygote) is produced. The zygote takes the form of a worm-like structure penetrating the stomach wall of the mosquito, forming a spherical cyst. Sporozoites are formed in great numbers throughout the mosquito's system including the salivary glands. Subsequent blood meals allow for the penetration of the parasite into other invertebrates. Within vertebrates asexual multiplication takes place in several phases. Subsequently red blood corpuscles are affected and malarial attacks result (from 48 to 72 hours in humans). Fever and chills result. The severity of these symptoms within humans varies depending upon the ecological parameters identified, and most severe cases are found in moist, tropical environments.

As explained by May, in order to develop an understanding of the ecological base of malaria it is necessary to examine the three-cycle interactance of parasite, vector, and human host. Climate, of course, plays an important role because certain kinds of anopheles are unable to survive in extremely cold environments, areas without sufficient moisture, and highland areas. In their study mentioned above, Dutta and Dutt have summarized malaria possibility in relation to temperatures in July and January (see Figure 41). In fact, the risk of malaria shifts with the angle of the sun and seasonal changes. Thus, during July the possibility of malaria shifts northward and during January the possibility shifts southward to include most land masses of the southern hemisphere. However, it should be pointed out that malaria eradication procedures over the last century have substantially reduced the threat of malaria in temperate and subtropical areas both north and south of the equator.

Geographers studying the ecology of malaria have taken several approaches. A recent study by Kovacik, for example, explains how the historical threat of malaria and various fevers in South Carolina contributed to the configuration and location of certain kinds of settlement, including resort areas.[29] South Carolina settlements were moved from coastal areas in reaction to perceived health hazards and amenities. The study by Dutta and Dutt pays some attention to the

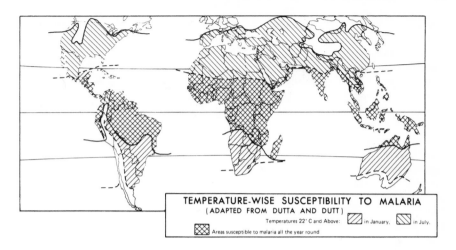

Fig. 41. Possibilities of Malaria susceptibility in relation to seasonality of temperature. Clearly, control measures have been implemented in most of the temperate climate areas.

incidence of malaria in relation to rainfall and relative humidity and explains how natural environmental elements have given rise to degrees of malaria incidence in Bengal. R. Mansell Prothero's research on migrants and malaria is an excellent case study of human activity in relation to disease. Prothero's detailed study explains how malaria can actually "migrate" with human populations engaged in various activities in some parts of the world, i.e., the disease moves with the host.[30] Yet another approach is exemplified by the studies of Learmonth[31] and Fonaroff[32] in analyses of natural environmental aspects of malaria, various kinds of human activity (particularly in relation to agricultural endeavors) and methods of detailed data acquisition.

The works of Learmonth and Fonaroff in the area of malaria geography are particularly important. Not only do they consider various aspects of the environment and human activity, but also take into account problems in terms of disease reporting and the results of eradication programs. Learmonth, for example, has offered information showing changes in malaria incidence as measured by human spleen rates in Mysore from 1928 to 1955. In that particular part of India, marked reductions in the incidence of malaria could be indicated through gradually decreasing spleen rates. Fonaroff's more detailed 1968 study shows similar results. His study of malaria in relation to agricultural activity, natural environmental factors and eradication programs details marked decreases in spleen rates in Trinidad from 1945 to 1950 and 1955 (see Figure 42). The contributions of Learmonth and Fonaroff have added to our knowledge of the

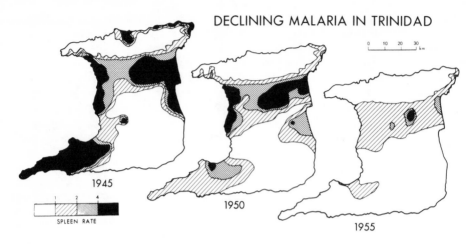

DECLINING MALARIA IN TRINIDAD

1945

1950

1955

SPLEEN RATE

Fig. 42. Fonoroff's explanation of declining Malaria in Trinidad from 1945 to 1955 on the basis of spleen rates.

geography of malaria and indicate a need for studies of changes in malaria distributions in particular areas by using large scale geographical analysis.

Such studies can make use of the findings of MacDonald.[33] He identified at least four major obstacles to malaria eradication in the mid-1960s. These included resistance to change due to certain kinds of human behavior, the resistance of some kinds of mosquitoes or parasites to control measures, the inability administratively to effect control programs, and a general inaccessibility of either people or mosquitoes to control measures. Control measures largely involve effective interruption of the transmission cycle of both the parasite and mosquitoes to forestall infection of humans. MacDonald indicated what may be a particular kind of geographical bias in relation to control programs by indicating a general lack of progress in Africa and the Eastern Mediterranean. While some progress has subsequently been made toward malaria control in certain parts of the Eastern Mediterranean, the greatest risks still appear to be in Africa. There is a rich literature in epidemiology on the mathematics of malaria transmission and control. In addition, geographers such as Learmonth and Fonaroff have made their contributions toward understanding environmental and cultural determinants of malaria. Additional progress toward malaria control and perhaps eradication can be made if these two approaches can be synthesized to a greater degree. Thus, specified case studies of environmental conditions combined with the mathematics of the epidemiology of the disease when outbreaks occur can lead to a better understanding of control. Since the disease is ubiquitous in so many specified environments, the complete elimination of malaria may be extremely difficult under current circumstances. If we are able to make malaria a disease of the past, then a breakthrough comparable to that accomplished with poliomyelitis may be necessary. It appears that nothing short of a vaccine may totally eliminate the disease, but, once again, the skills of the medical geographer can be applied more than at present.

Yet another disease wherein much is known of both the ecology of the disease in relation to geographical factors as well as the mathematics of the epidemiology is human schistosomiasis, or *Bilharziasis*. Human schistosomiasis is a chronic endemic disease particularly affecting the liver, intestine, and bladder of victims and often causing long-term debilitation. Farooq's account of the history of the disease explains how schistosomiasis was known in ancient Mesopotamia and Egypt.[34] As early as 1900 B.C., hieroglyphics gave indications of human symptoms of schistosomiasis and curative practices at that time. Much of our present-day knowledge of general factors responsible for the endemicity and propagation of this disease date to the turn of this century. It is now known that at least three major forms of the disease, *Schistosoma mansoni, S. haematobium,* and *S. japonicum* are distributed in different parts of the world. The presence of *S. mansoni* in the new world was specifically identified by Priaja da Silva in 1904 in Brazil. *S. japonicum* was studied during the 19th century, and the first concrete evidence of the causative agent of the disease was recorded by Katsurada, also in 1904. By the end of World War II, particularly through the efforts of Leiper, valuable information contributed to understanding *S. haematobium.* The term schistosomiasis can generally be applied to several kinds of interrelated diseases involving several species as well as strains of parasites. One common element is that life cycles are very similar (see Figure 43).[35]

LIFE CYCLE OF SCHISTOSOMA MANSONI

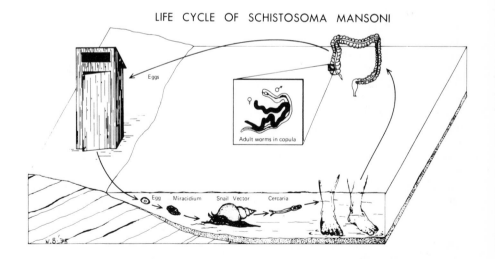

Fig. 43. The life cycle of Schistosoma mansoni.

Schistosomiasis is caused by atypical trematodes (flat worms) manifesting life cycles in the following stages: egg, miracidium, two generations of sporocyst, cercaria, and adult. In man, clinical forms of the disease are vesical and intestinal. Vesical forms are caused by *S. haematobium* and intestinal forms by *S. mansoni* and *S. japonicum*. The actual infection is casued by the cercaria. It is possible for a man to enter the cycle of schistosomiasis infection primarily through activities associated with an aquatic medium, providing the opportunity for cercarial infection. Such activities include caring for aquatic animals, washing clothing, swimming, wading, farming, or any other reasons requiring entry into relatively still waters. The free-swimming cercaria invade the human body by perforation of the skin. This is not the only manner of ingestion as a much more rapid schistosomiasis infection can result from drinking contaminated water. Even with penetration the process is relatively fast, averaging approximately three minutes. For *mansoni* infections the parasite passes through the heart and lungs and enters the liver wherein male and female adult worms pair. The habitat of *japonicum* is basically the mesenteric veins and for *haematobium* it is in the bladder and pelvic areas. Eggs are produced from the paired adults and leave the human system either through the feces or the urinary tract. The eggs do not hatch until they reach the aquatic medium and the miracidium emerges.

Clinical and pathological aspects of schistosomiasis in humans can be manifested by coughing, sometimes accompanied by viscous mucus or blood and at other times bronchial asthma. In general, the disease has a debilitating effect and is sometimes manifested by early symptoms which may appear to be related to bacterial or viral infections followed by diarrhea, weakness, and fever. There is a progressive degeneration associated with schistosome infections leading to a sort of congestive syndrome caused by the body's reactions to the presence of foreign matter. In some instances there is a characteristic enlargement of the liver and spleen. Strength of the victim is substantially lowered and in many instances resistance to other forms of infection is substantially reduced. In the early 1970s, Wright estimated that there may have been as many as 125,000,000 persons infected by schistosomiasis throughout the world.[36] It was further estimated that more than 90 million persons in Africa were infected, another 25 million in Southeast Asis, and more than 6 million in the Americas.

As part of its long-term efforts to control schistosomiasis, the World Health Organization has provided information pertaining to the distribution of various types of schistosomiasis affecting human beings throughout the world. In addition, the following authors have studied the worldwide distribution of schistosomiasis: Hunter, Schwartzwelder, and Clyde; Faust; Marcial-Rojas; and Wright.[37] The pattern shown within Figure 44 is a synthesis of the distributional mapping accomplished by these researchers and the World Health Organization. For example, *S. mansoni* has been identified to be particularly prevalent in parts of the Antilles, Venezuela, parts of northeast Brazil and scattered pockets throughout the southern part of West Africa, eastern Africa, and Madagascar. *S. japonicum* is distributed primarily in parts of Japan, the Philippines, Southeast Asia, the West Indies, and extensive parts of China, and *S. haematobium* follows distributional patterns similar to those of *S. mansoni* in Africa but has been

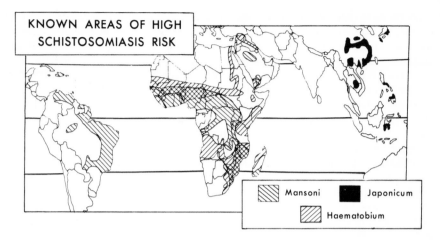

Fig. 44. Known areas of high Schistosomiasis risk for three major types.

identified to be particularly prevalent in the Middle East, Egypt, Sudan, and Ethiopia. Many of the differences in distributions of various types of schistosomiasis are directly related to the presence of different kinds of intermediate snail hosts.

While a general statement can be made that the three major types of schistosomiasis affecting human beings can be found in specified tropical and subtropical parts of the world, there are general juxtapositions of environmental circumstances which help explain the optimum conditions for the overall transmission cycle of schistosomiasis. These factors include altitude, temperature, oxygen tension, light, gravity, rainfall, water movement, salinity, dissolved oxygen, vegetation, and of course the presence of man near the water.[38] Since the snails feed on particular kinds of vegetation near the surface of either slow-moving or relatively stagnant waters, the miracidium are attracted to the surface and the intermediate snail hosts. It has been pointed out that bottom dwelling gastropods are not nearly so attractive to the miracidium as those dwelling near the surface. Temperature also influences the life cycles of these parasites and ranges of from 5 to 40°C are generally understood as the parameters for the three major types of schistosomiasis transmission. Temperatures, of course, are influenced in tropical and subtropical areas by altitude. Light definitely plays a role because of the feeding habits of snails near the surface of water and the growth of vegetation. While rainfall is essential to the survival of schistosome eggs, insufficient or excessive rainfall contributing to water turbulence both decrease the possibilities of schistosomiasis. General salinity also is a factor because excessive salt content in the water may inhibit the process of egg hatching. Human activity as part of the total environment contributes to infection in several ways. A major source of transmission consists of human pollution of water and the placement of latrines and similar disposal stations too close to the kind of water amenable to the schistosomiasis cycle. Haddock's case study of *Schistosomiasis mansoni* in Puerto Rico has been used here to explain the complexities of the disease problem in more detail.

The diffusion of *S. mansoni* into the Americas has generally been associated with the importation of African slaves, particularly in the West Indies and Brazil. It is estimated that there are in excess of 200,000 cases of schistosomiasis in Puerto Rico. The physiographic configuration of Puerto Rico is somewhat complex and leads to concentrations of the disease in certain parts of the island (see Figure 45). The island is dominated by a central mountain system with few extensive plains. The heaviest rainfall is in the northeastern part of the island with lesser amounts in the south and west. Since rainfall is seasonal, it is during the drier seasons when waters are more still that snail populations and aquatic vegetation are established in certain streams, generally with a gradient of less than 2%. In Haddock's study of Puerto Rico, he paid particular attention to the snail *B. glabrata.* Conditions for breeding this particular snail are largely met in the wet eluvial parts of Puerto Rico north of the central mountains and in the eastern part of the island. Some snails have also been found in areas under irrigation on the southern coast. In 1968 Ferguson pointed out that schistosomiasis is not only distributed somewhat unevenly within Puerto Rico, but it is also an urban and suburban disease as well as one of more severity in rural

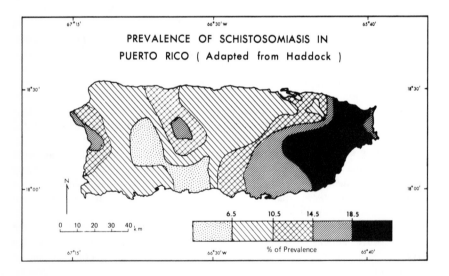

Fig. 45. An adaptation of Haddock's explanation of the prevalence of Schistosomiasis in Puerto Rico.

parts of the country.[39] He also found that in spite of seasonality in rainfall that repopulation was quite rapid and a colony of snails could be revitalized within a few months.

According to MacDonald, in his studies of the probability of schistosomiasis infections, four major types of treatment can be used in the process.[40] The most effective appears to be chemotherapy, although there is some controversy pertaining to the use of drug treatment. In addition, control of snail populations and control of water flows have also worked. A fourth method is sanitation control. In an analysis of a decade and a half of schistosomiasis control in selected parts of Puerto Rico, Jobin, Ferguson, and Palmer reported in 1970 that control of snail populations proved quite effective, although it was learned later that chemotherapy programs had been initiated throughout Puerto Rico at the same time.[41] The particular area of study used by the above authors included sugar cane raising locations in the southern part of Puerto Rico.[42] In testing a sample of 6 year-olds for schistosomiasis, Jobin, Ferguson, and Palmer found that over a period of time, snail control was indeed quite effective in reducing schistosomiasis. Additional reports from St. Lucia on a project initiated in 1965 by the government of St. Lucia and the Rockefeller Foundation focusing on alterations in mechanisms supplying household water report some progress in that experimental control measure.[43] Unrau reported via the World Health Organization in 1975 that improvements in water supplies could control *S. mansoni.*[44] In another study by Jordan, Woodstock, Unrau, and Cook, also from the St. Lucia project, it was contended that the intensity of infection with *S. mansoni* was significantly reduced because of improvements of household water supplies.[45]

The literature on control of schistosomiasis is nearly as extensive as that identifying the disease problem. On the subject of chemotherapy, for example, Peter Jordan explains that one primary objective is to stop the dissemination of eggs in infected human beings.[46] There appear to be little differences in therapeutic responses to available drugs because the treatments are egg growth suppressors rather than cures at this time. There also have been some side effects reported. Jordan suggests a combined effort including those aspects suggested by MacDonald, i.e., chemotherapy, water control, snail control, and sanitation. Many attempts to eradicate snails have been reported. Many experimental projects consist of controlled studies in specific sites where water flows are altered, snails are identified, and a variety of chemicals are used to develop better methods of controlling snail populations. There are, of course, certain ecological problems which can affect other aquatic life in this process, but efforts in many parts of the world are now being carried on with the aim of control in mind. While there is no "cure" at this time, research is also taking place trying to develop an understanding of measures necessary to develop a vaccine.

Schistosomiasis and malaria have been identified as two major parasitic diseases of the world today. Different control measures in different parts of the world have resulted in a variety of prevalence reductions. In the case of malaria it is absolutely necessary to maintain as many control measures as possible as the disease will flare up. Studies of schistosomiasis control have been extremely intensive and until such time that a vaccine might possibly be developed, the same holds true for that disease. For both diseases environmental factors play such an important role that geographic aspects of the disease ecology must constantly be kept in mind and perhaps considered as part of interdisciplinary efforts to conquer these diseases. Even in developed nations, geographic aspects of the ecology of human disease are necessary to formulate control measures. The following two North American examples are offered as case studies.

CASE STUDIES IN DISEASE ECOLOGY:
NORTH AMERICAN EXAMPLES

The schistosomiasis saga indicates how knowledge about disease transmission can be greatly enhanced by studying associations with natural environmental conditions using the disease ecological approach. Some have criticized many of these analyses as too retrospective in nature, and the problem of schistosomiasis is far from solved. We know of such geographic factors as climate, drainage, and human use of periodically flooded agricultural areas contributing to the spread of schistosomiasis. And these factors have been studied intensely. We have known of the problem in Egypt. In addition, recent information pertaining to an increase of schistosomiasis in the Sudan plus Soviet redefinitions of schistosomiasis areas within Ethiopia are to some extend disheartening. This disappointment is primarily due to the fact that even the knowledge of environmental aspects leading to disease hazard the disease problems cannot be halted unless there is response in the form of governmental action leading to control. This problem is by no means restricted to more tropical or subtropical parts of the world. It is simply that these areas have been studied more intensely. Disease ecological approaches, including public policy ramifications of the identification of environmental risk factors, can be explored within more temperate parts of the world and in areas that are considered parts of modern industrial society. Following Knight's suggestion that we perhaps best understand arthropod-borne diseases within the context of disease ecological approaches, two examples, California encephalitis and Rocky Mountain spotted fever in the United States during recent times, are used. Vectored infectious diseases are by no means restricted to more tropical, "backward" or isolated parts of the earth.

Arthropod-Borne Encephalitis

In epidemiological studies it is common practice at the discovery of many disease-causing agents to name particular diseases after locations where they have initially been isolated. One kind of mosquito-borne encephalitis, now widely accepted as California encephalitis, is now known to be part of a larger interrelated group of viruses affecting humans. Venezuelan, West Nile, Simliki Forest, Bunyamwera, Ntaya, Japanese B, Russian Spring–Summer, Eastern, Western, St. Louis, LaCrosse, and California are all names which have been used. In different parts of the world it is expected that different names would be used for variations of arthropod-borne encephalitis characterized by similar symptoms in humans. Clearly, not all species of mosquitos are widespread throughout the world. Still, important aspects of arthropod-borne encephalitis include generally similar environmental conditions which can be studied within the context of medical geography.

Geographic studies of arthropod-borne encephalitis are difficult to pursue for a variety of reasons. One problem is that isolations have been made in scattered locations, and different names have been given to similar sets of symptoms. Also, there are several kinds of encephalitis affecting humans. Some forms of this inflammation of the brain may be due to injury or complications following some other infectious disease, mumps or measles for example. Symptoms in humans vary and some cases are not severe. Included among these symptoms might be headache, nausea, vomiting, fever, sore throat, chills, stiff neck, drowsiness, trembling, vertigo, convulsions, and possibly coma. Given modern treatment methods, few persons actually die from encephalitis; a more serious problem consists of serious aftereffects including retardation, paralysis or even mental instability. There is, unfortunately, now no vaccine for immunization and the best method of treatment consists of the use of antibiotics.

Given knowledge of geographic factors contributing to the disease, it can also be controlled by limiting the proliferation of particular kinds of mosquitos in areas identified endemic to arthropod-borne encephalitis.[47] Methodological developments within the past 25 years in medical geography and medical knowledge about arthropod-borne encephalitis can be combined to study the disease problem. The following four steps can be utilized by a researcher in accomplishing such a task: (1) the identification of biogeographic aspects of mosquito-borne encephalitis common to diverse locations; (2) the study of common aspects of environments which appear to be contributing to excessive amounts of arthropod-borne encephalitis; (3) on the basis of generalized mapping develop more detailed scale identifications of endemic areas; and (4) identify specific environmental risk hazards within endemic areas and compare these areas for evidence of common environmental problems.

The identification of encephalitis virus is a good example of the use of general geographic information in many ways. For a period of approximately 30 years (1933 to 1964), unique yet related viruses were investigated within a variety of locations in the United States and other parts of the world. Areas known to have encephalitis problems were selected as locations for the establishment of laboratories. The identification of what has become known as California encephalitis was first published in substantial detail in the early 1950s, although information had been gradually accumulating since the early 1930s.[48] Hammond, Reeves, and Sather reported the isolation of encephalitis virus from *Aedes dorsalis* and *Culex tarsalis* mosquitos in their now well-known 1952 study of the San Joaquin Valley of California.[49] Laboratory techniques included the use of small mammals, domestic fowl, horses, and wild birds for evidence of encephalitis virus isolated in mosquitos and humans. It was concluded that a variety of intermediate hosts could be identified, particularly the mosquito-wild-bird-mosquito virus life cycle and to some extent small mammals as intermediate hosts. Eventually, epidemiological researchers were to make the statement that arthropod-borne encephalitis was "widespread geographically."[50]

During the 1950s and early 1960s studies of arthropod-borne encephalitis virus increased. A related virus was recovered from a snowshoe hare in Montana in 1955, and in 1958 a similar virus was recovered in Czechoslovakia and termed Tahyna.[51] It was evident within the United States by the mid-1960s that a complex interrelationship between several kinds of encephalitis virus, for example, LaCrosse and California, recurred continuously in seriologic studies within different parts of the country. By 1964 a complex California encephalitis group was well known.[52] Epidemiological studies had associated the disease generally with environments akin to more natural habitats and to farm areas. In many instances horses and barnyard fowl were identified as having similar encephalitis characteristics. Wild birds and small mammals normally inhabiting temperate forests were tested and found to be immune carriers. Combinations of such environmental conditions as presence of woodlands, areas with poor drainage, and places with periodic cycles of rainfall were considered to be somehow contributing to outbreaks of California encephalitis in humans.

During the several decades of identification of California encephalitis few cases were reported either to state departments of health or to the Communicable Disease Center in Atlanta, Georgia. After 1964, however, when the California group was better known, reporting did increase. Of particular importance was knowledge of the relationship between the LaCrosse virus first identified in Wisconsin and the general California group. The LaCrosse strain was subsequently identified in horses in a semirural part of southeastern Pennsylvania, and in 1964 several kinds of mosquitos were discovered to be carriers of California encephalitis in Ohio.[53] One particular location in Ohio, the village of Gambier, was considered to be endemic; and detailed epidemiological field studies of the area attributed the high rates of California encephalitis to several environmental phenomena. Mosquito proliferation was explained by the presence of a mixed mesophtic forest including a particular kind of Silver Maple that seemed to attract mosquitos. It was also implied that glaciation of the area contributed to poor drainage conditions allowing for many locations where mosquitos could breed. Also, it was noted that farm animals were found in the area immediately surrounding the small village. Figure 46 is adapted from an epidemiological field map of the Gambier, Ohio area constructed by Dr. Richard Berry and his colleagues investigating the encephalitis problem. The black dots show the distribution of human California encephalitis cases from 1964 to 1971 in the Gambier area. Note the number of cases in areas of mixed forest.

The epidemiological field map constructed by Bardos and Danielova in Czechoslovakia more than a decade earlier than Berry and his colleagues shows some interesting environmental similarities. Bardos and Danielova selected a study area in the southern portion of East Slovakia; a lowland area known to have a high mosquito population. There were farms in the area and numerous rivers contributed to periodic flooding and the development of poorly drained areas (see Figure 47). The assumption was made that circulation of the virus among wild and domestic animals could be identified in relation to the geography of the area. In addition, this part of East Slovakia is in the path of migratory birds possibly contributing to wintering-over of the virus. An encephalitis virus was

KNOX COUNTY, OHIO

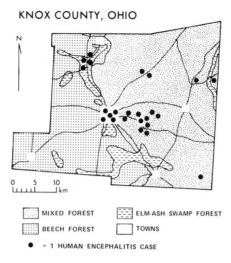

MIXED FOREST ▨ ELM-ASH SWAMP FOREST

BEECH FOREST ☐ TOWNS

● = 1 HUMAN ENCEPHALITIS CASE

Fig. 46. Human Encephalitis cases in Knox County, Ohio in relation to natural ecological conditions.

TAHYNA AREA OF CZECHOSLOVAKIA

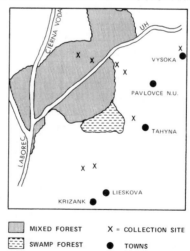

▨ MIXED FOREST   X = COLLECTION SITE

▨ SWAMP FOREST   ● TOWNS

Fig. 47. The Tahyna area of Czechoslovakia where mosquitos carrying the Encephalitis virus were captured. Note the proximity of swamp and mixed forest.

identified from mosquitos trapped near the village of Tahyna. Although large numbers of mosquitos were tested in relation to the number of positive isolations, they had the most success when examining mosquitos found in farm sheds. The most important aspect of this study was that encephalitis virus were identified in *Aedes caspius,* a kind of mosquito closely related to *Aedes dorsalis,* one species later to be known as an encephalitis carrier in the United States.

Comparing Figures 46 and 47, several questions might be posed pertaining to what these areas have in common. One aspect that stands out in both studies is the information about excessive mosquito populations due to poor drainage and proximity to mixed forests. Following this environmental "clue" it is possible to examine this hypothesis further. Cases of confirmed California encephalitis reported in the state of Ohio from 1964 to 1975 have been shown to cluster in areas within and adjacent to floodplains (see Figure 48). The large cluster between Columbus and Mansfield is in the Knox County area. When a comparison was made between the temporal distribution of cases of confirmed California encephalitis and rainfall in endemic areas, it was discovered that disease outbreaks follow summer rains. Figure 49 shows the distribution of these confirmed cases during the time period 1964 to 1975. There was early reporting in the spring and a gradual increase during the months of June, July, and August with a peak in September. Reporting then fell with decreasing temperatures. A comparison was made with rainfall peaks, and it was found that a lag ranging from one to two weeks could be identified between the time that rainfall peaked and encephalitis reporting increased. This complex environmental association consists of California encephalitis endemicity within parts of the state, accumulation of water following rain in poorly drained areas adjacent to the epidemic areas, the increased breeding of mosquitos, and the transmission of California encephalitis to humans. Intermediate hosts, such as wild or domestic mammals or birds, may or may not be involved in this transmission cycle.

A detailed examination of the distribution of some confirmed cases of California encephalitis within the Akron, Ohio area (considered endemic) explains how natural environmental factors also contribute to arthropod-borne encephalitis in an urban industrialized area. The Akron area is on a drainage divide between waters flowing into Lake Erie and the Ohio River. Previous glaciation in the area caused substantial disruptions in former drainage patterns and the development of many glacial lakes and poorly drained areas. In the northwestern part of the city, the valley of the Cuyahoga River is fairly wide and somewhat deep for that particular part of the state. In addition, the floodplain of an older stream is contained within a larger valley. Parts of the valley are wooded and ravines draining into the Cuyahoga River Valley form portions of a metropolitan park. Figure 50 shows the distribution of confirmed cases of California encephalitis in relation to the ravines and wooded areas. Epidemiological field studies indicated that mosquitos were no doubt breeding in the floodplain below the populated portion of this area. Somehow the California encephalitis virus was carried up the floodplain into the settled area to cause infection in some children. Perhaps the mosquito-wild bird-mosquito association was involved. Perhaps wild mammals were involved. On the other hand, perhaps there was no

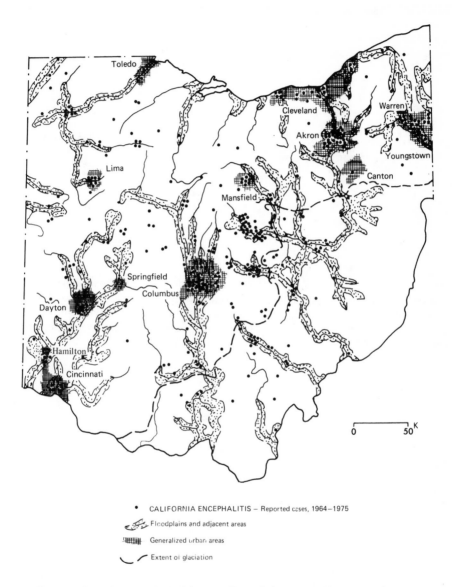

● CALIFORNIA ENCEPHALITIS – Reported cases, 1964–1975

Floodplains and adjacent areas

Generalized urban areas

Extent of glaciation

Fig. 48. Prevalence of California Encephalitis in Ohio in relation to floodplains and settled areas.

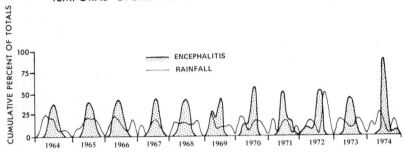

Fig. 49. A comparison of cycles of Encephalitis and rainfall in endemic parts of Ohio. Note that most of the time Encephalitis cycles are followed by seasonal rainfall patterns.

intermediate host. The important point in this particular microscale geographical analysis is that environmental factors contributing to the spread of California encephalitis were uncovered. By selectively spraying the floodplain below the settled area and portions of the metropolitan park, the problem of California encephalitis was brought under control.

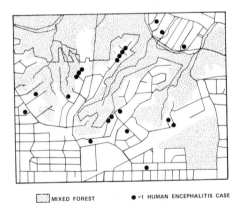

MIXED FOREST   ● =1 HUMAN ENCEPHALITIS CASE

Fig. 50. Distribution of Encephalitis cases within part of Akron, Ohio in relation to an area of ravines and mixed forest adjacent to settled areas.

The disease still has epidemic potential within the Akron area as well as several other portions of the state of Ohio. Control of the disease is also a problem of timing. The most effective spraying programs are those which occur immediately after the peaks of rainfall. However, this peak cannot be determined in advance and the best measures are to continue to spray in poorly drained areas with floodplain-like characteristics if the disease is to be controlled. What is not known is how the disease winters over since the virus cannot live without a host. There is speculation that it might winter over in domestic pigeons as well as small mammals. One interesting theory is the possibility that it actually winters over in warmer climates within the red-winged blackbird, known to be an encephalitis virus carrier, and the virus is annually returned to the state via these birds. This kind of transmission possibility is suggested as an area of further research in medical geography.

In a different kind of encephalitis study, two Soviet researchers, Birulya and Zalutskaya, demonstrated in 1967 that certain kinds of environmental factors may be related to tick-borne encephalitis within the Soviet Union.[54] In their particular analysis they uncovered what they identified as a five-factor environmental complex associated with the development of tick-borne encephalitis. These factors consisted of climate, landforms, plant cover, the identification of tick hosts, and what they termed secondary landscapes within the Soviet Union. In general, optimal conditions for the formation of tick infestation foci seemed to arise in those parts of the Soviet Union shown as the darkest areas within Figure 51. While natural infestation of animals is common, in environments subject to the greatest amount of disruption of natural conditions, tick infestation has proved to be a greater problem with humans. While this particular kind of generalization at the national scale is of limited utility, the notion of disruption of the natural environment and proliferation of tick-borne diseases is of particular importance in studies of disease ecology.

Disease Ecological Aspects of Rocky Mountain Spotted Fever

Rocky Mountain spotted fever is one of several kinds of tick-borne fevers belonging to the rickettsial disease group. According to Imperato, there are four kinds of tick-borne spotted fever recognized internationally.[55] In the United States, Canada, Panama, Mexico, and South America, Rocky Mountain spotted fever (caused by *Rickettsia rickettsii*) is spread to humans by bites from ticks. Wild rodents and domestic dogs are the most widespread recognized reservoirs. The incubation period for Rocky Mountain spotted fever is from 3 to 14 days. In Africa, India, Europe, and the Middle East *Rickettsia conori* has been described as the agent causing related Boutonneuse fever. Ticks also serve as vectors; rodents and dogs act as reservoirs. This kind of fever has an incubation of from 5 to 7 days. In Australia, particularly Queensland, tick typhus caused by *Rickettsia australia* and, again, involving ticks and rodents has an incubation period of from 7 to 10 days. In the Soviet Union and Mongolia, Siberian tick typhus with *Rickettsia siberica* recognized as an agent is transmitted in a similar fashion. This particular disease has the most limited incubation period, lasting

INFECTION FOCI OF TICK—BORNE ENCEPHALITIS AND LANDFORMS

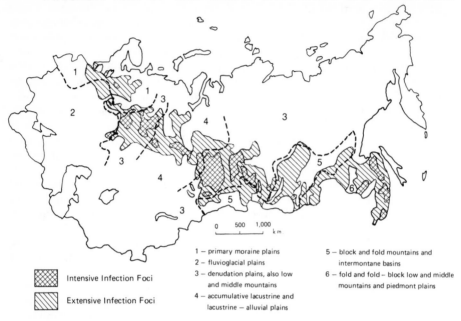

Intensive Infection Foci

Extensive Infection Foci

1 — primary moraine plains

2 — fluvioglacial plains

3 — denudation plains, also low and middle mountains

4 — accumulative lacustrine and lacustrine — alluvial plains

5 — block and fold mountains and intermontane basins

6 — fold and fold — block low and middle mountains and piedmont plains

Fig. 51. General locations within the Soviet Union with natural ecological conditions contributing to the possibility of Tick-borne Encephalitis.

from 2 to 7 days. Survival from any of these four kinds of spotted fever normally results in immunity. In the case of Rocky Mountain spotted fever, a vaccine is available.

Symptoms of Rocky Mountain spotted fever generally include the rapid onset of a high fever, sometimes within a few days in severe cases, a skin rash and headache.[56] Other symptoms include loss of appetite, malaise, sometimes chilly sensations, and a particularly characteristic rash. The classic Rocky Mountain spotted fever rash initially appears on ankles and wrists and spreads to the remainder of the body. The rash may appear anywhere from the second to the sixth day. Some complications can unfortunately result from Rocky Mountain spotted fever. These include pneumonia, hemorrhages, acute nephritis, impaired hearing or sight, and anemia.

Knowledge of geographic factors contributing to the proliferation of Rocky Mountain spotted fever in the United States is of importance to public health workers searching for improved control measures. Terrain and natural vegetation conditions appear to combine in certain ways to form ecological "niches" suitable for this particular disease in a natural state. It was initially thought to be more prevalent in wooded highland locations. Recently cases have been reported with greater frequency in more settled locations along the eastern piedmont of the United States. Land use change in rural areas and suburban expansion may be contributing to sufficient disruption of natural habitats in such a manner that this change is taking place. Rocky Mountain spotted fever is of particular research interest in medical geography because we may have one of the few examples in recent times of a disease which has probably undergone relocation diffusion.

Historical accounts identify this disease as definitely endemic to the Rocky Mountain portions of the United States. During this century endemic areas of Rocky Mountain spotted fever have shifted from the western to the eastern United States. There are differing theories, however, in terms of whether the disease has actually gone through relocation diffusion in terms of geographic endemicity or simply that control of the disease in the west and better recognition of the disease in the east has in fact shifted the geographic foci of the disease. Different researchers have different theories regarding the reasons for this presumed shift. Regardless of the reasons, Rocky Mountain spotted fever is definitely most endemic in the eastern piedmont sections of the United States, in the Appalachians, and in parts of Oklahoma. Figure 52 shows reported cases in 1976.

ROCKY MOUNTAIN SPOTTED FEVER—Reported Cases by County, 1976

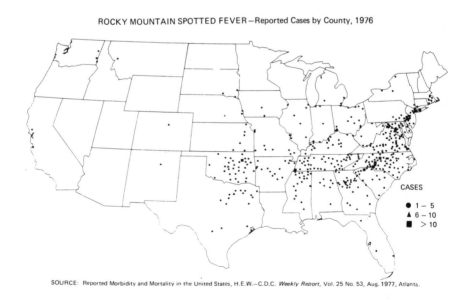

SOURCE: Reported Morbidity and Mortality in the United States, H.E.W.–C.D.C. *Weekly Report*, Vol. 25 No. 53, Aug. 1977, Atlanta.

Fig. 52. The reporting of Rocky Mountain Spotted Fever in the United States in 1976.

Rocky Mountain spotted fever was first formally described in the late 19th century. In 1906 Ricketts offered proof that the disease was spread by *Dermacentor andersoni,* the wood tick. Until the 1930s the disease was thought to be limited to the western United States. At that time, however, researchers recognized clinically similar symptoms in certain eastern seaboard states. It was further discovered that the eastern dog tick (*Dermacentor variabilis*) was a major vector in spreading the disease in that part of the country. With the development of a vaccine and the subsequent use of broad range antibiotic treatment, the incidence of Rocky Mountain spotted fever declined during the 1940s and 1950s. The disease continued to decline through the 1950s to reach a low point in the early 1960s. It has been steadily on the increase since 1960, and the shift in reporting from western to eastern states is well known.

In a 1964 study, Atwood, Lamb, and Sonenshine examined the ecology of Rocky Mountain spotted fever in the eastern United States, paying particular attention to the problem in the state of Virginia.[57] They examined the ecology of the disease in relation to physiographic provinces, trends in land use change and natural vegetation. They found that during 1960 and 1961 case rates in Virginia were highest in the piedmont area, second highest in the coastal plain, and third highest in more mountainous parts of the state. There were more rural than urban cases and more suburban cases than urban. Abandoned fields and wooded areas, particularly in the piedmont, appeared to be likely geographic locations for the breeding of ticks. They attributed this possibility to secondary tree growth and the possible proliferation of brush type plants. Along with other hypotheses, aspects of land use change rated high on their list. Also, many victims of Rocky Mountain spotted fever in the eastern part of the United States tended to be younger and there was a higher proportion of infected females than had been reported earlier in the western United States. The western version in part showed a higher incidence of victims engaged in such occupations as logging and a variety of summer outdoor activities. In other words, the ecology of "western" Rocky Mountain spotted fever was much more classic in its dependency on wild habitats than the eastern version. Sonenshine continued to work with other researchers through the 1970s in developing an understanding of the natural ecology of Rocky Mountain spotted fever in the eastern United States. In a 1970 study, for example, Rothenberg and Sonenshine explained that from 1960 to 1963 large proportions of those contracting Rocky Mountain spotted fever in Virginia were students, preschool children, and housewives.[58] Fewer cases were reported by construction workers, surveyors, and pest control workers, with intermediate numbers reported by farmers.

In 1972, Sonenshine, Peters, and Levy compared Rocky Mountain spotted fever with natural vegetation patterns in the eastern United States for the two decade period from 1951 to 1971.[59] They examined the geographic distribution of Rocky Mountain spotted fever in the eastern United States (a pattern very similar to Figure 52) and compared the disease distribution to maps showing natural vegetation types. They proved through use of a chi-square test that the distribution of cases of Rocky Mountain spotted fever were significantly different from random. They then put forth an hypothesis that high concentrations of the disease were found in the hickory-pine forest belt of the eastern United States. Additional significant associations were found in the oak-hickory-pine forest areas. They further explored distributions of tick vectors and offered evidence to further support the contention that the vector of Rocky Mountain spotted fever in the eastern United States is the dog tick.

Sonenshine and his colleagues showed some disagreement with an hypothesis set forth in 1959 by Smadel that the changing process of urbanization was having an influence on changing patterns of Rocky Mountain spotted fever.[60] Smadel's hypothesis deserves attention in light of what has occurred since the 1950s because the statement was made when Rocky Mountain spotted fever was at an all time low in the United States. Recent investigations have shown that population shifts and land use change can contribute to changing patterns of Rocky Mountain spotted fever reporting. The information provided by Sonenshine and his colleagues pertaining to the breeding potential of natural vegetation can be viewed as positive evidence of the natural ecological factors contributing to the disease in conjunction with population change. In many instances when locations with potential Rocky Mountain spotted fever endemicity change from wild areas to suburban areas, or from farms to overgrown areas, certain kinds of birds or mammals serving as reservoirs of the disease may either leave or reinhabit areas. Increased urban growth and suburbanization also mean pets, dogs and cats particularly. Both of these mammals serve as excellent reservoirs for the disease. From a geographic point of view, the natural ecological explanations of Sonenshine and his colleagues are not at odds with the population change hypothesis of Smadel. An analysis of Rocky Mountain spotted fever in South Carolina helps explain this statement.

During the summer of 1977 a geographical analysis of patterns of Rocky Mountain spotted fever distributions in South Carolina was initiated by Pyle. Some preliminary results are discussed here. Information was obtained from the state of South Carolina, Department of Health and Environmental Control, for all confirmed cases of Rocky Mountain spotted fever reported for the time period 1966 through 1976.[61] Initially, a Poisson probability map was developed on the basis of that information (see discussion of McGlashan's use of this method in chapter 3). The resultant pattern is contained within Figure 53. The darkest areas are those parts of the state with the highest percent probability that reporting of Rocky Mountain spotted fever is not due to chance. Other areas show lesser probabilities. It is not surprising to find that the parts of South Carolina with the highest probability of significant reporting are commonly referred to as "up country." Reference to the topographic profile within Figure 53 indicates these areas as the piedmont and foothills to the Appalachians. These parts of South Carolina contain the natural ecological conditions explained by Sonenshine and others. It is also of interest that this section of South Carolina has demonstrated increased population growth during the period of investigation.

On the basis of the statewide Poisson probabilities, 5 counties within South Carolina (Anderson, Greenville, Pickens, Spartanburg, and York) were selected for more detailed analysis. Figure 54 contains the distribution of settled places in those counties. Four of the 5 counties have experienced increased growth over

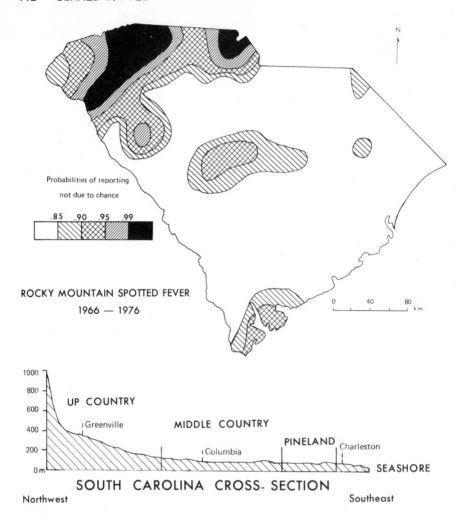

ROCKY MOUNTAIN SPOTTED FEVER
1966 — 1976

Probabilities of reporting
not due to chance

.85   .90   .95   .99

UP COUNTRY

Greenville

MIDDLE COUNTRY

Columbia

PINELAND   Charleston

SEASHORE

SOUTH CAROLINA CROSS- SECTION

Northwest   Southeast

Fig. 53. Areas of Rocky Mountain Spotted Fever concentration in South Carolina from 1966 to 1976.

the past decade. York County, the exception, should demonstrate some growth once Interstate Highway 77 is completed from Rock Hill to Columbia, the state capitol.

Figure 55 shows locations of Rocky Mountain spotted fever cases reported from 1966 to 1976 within each of these counties in relation to land use.[62] In almost every instance there are higher numbers of reported cases in urbanized

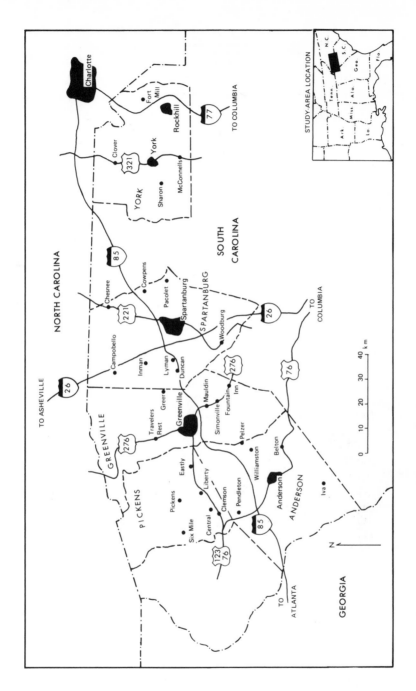

Fig. 54. Counties in the northern part of South Carolina where Rocky Mountain Spotted Fever is prevalent.

113

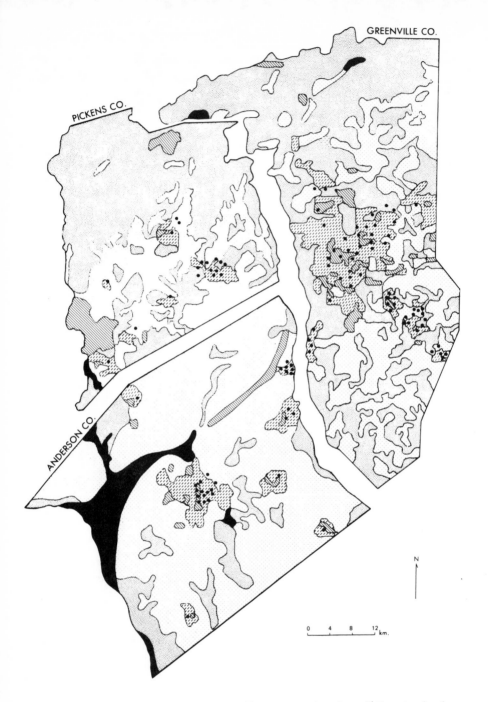

Fig. 55. Rocky Mountain Spotted Fever reporting in relation to land use patterns. *Part 1.*

114

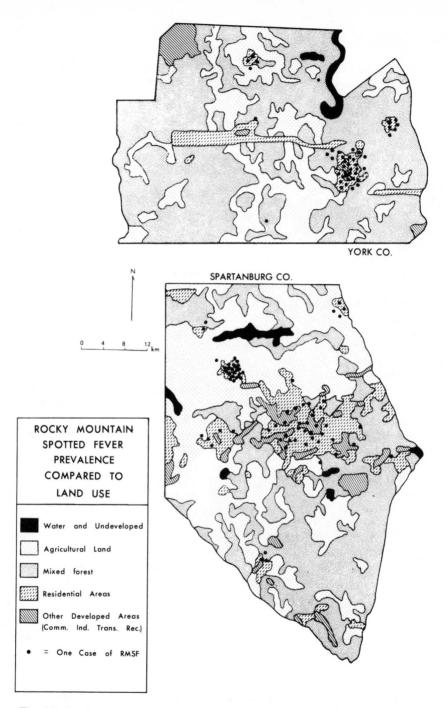

YORK CO.

SPARTANBURG CO.

N

0   4   8   12
                km

ROCKY MOUNTAIN
SPOTTED FEVER
PREVALENCE
COMPARED TO
LAND USE

■ Water and Undeveloped

□ Agricultural Land

▨ Mixed forest

▨ Residential Areas

▨ Other Developed Areas
    (Comm. Ind. Trans. Rec.)

• = One Case of RMSF

Fig. 55. Rocky Mountain Spotted Fever reporting in relation to land use patterns. *Part 2.*

and suburbanized parts of the counties than in more rural and forested parts of the counties. Chi-square tests were performed for each county comparing rural and urban areas and incidence above and below the average reporting. In every instance the hypothesis that the distribution of reported cases of Rocky Mountain spotted fever is not related to developed parts of the counties was rejected.

Examination of growth patterns in relation to the incidence of reported cases within the counties generally substantiates Smadel's hypothesis of almost 20 years ago. For example, in Anderson County, the city of Anderson showed a 4.9% increase in population from 1966 to 1976.[63] Iva, a settlement reporting one case, showed a 6% population loss. Conversely, Pelzer, a town with a 5.5% increase in growth, had concentrations of cases. Interstate Highway 85 was completed during this time period, thus opening this part of the "Sunbelt" to migration of industry and ultimately population from other places. This kind of growth produces suburbanization and subsequent disruption of otherwise natural habitats and suggests the replacement of wild mammals with household pets as reservoirs of Rocky Mountain spotted fever. A similar association can be made within Greenville County; however, in this instance the largest settlement, Greenville, with the most reporting of spotted fever did show a 5% population loss during this time period. Settlements with significant reporting of spotted fever and substantial population growth in Greenville County included Maldin, Simpsonville, and Fountain Inn. When similar comparisons are made for Spartanburg, Pickins, and parts of York Counties, a direct relationship can generally be made between population increase and the intensity of reporting of Rocky Mountain spotted fever. In the case of Spartanburg County, the development of Interstate Highways 26 and 85 have ultimately contributed to improved transportation accessibility and general overall growth, and, indirectly, the disease problem.

During the summers of 1977 and 1978, reporting of the disease continued to increase in many of the locations shown within Figure 53. In South Carolina, the number of cases reported has remained about the same for the last several years (1975 to 1978) in spite of increase elsewhere. The most effective control strategy appears to be public education. Teams of public health workers regularly visit endemic locations and explain the disease problem to school children, groups of employees in extractive industries, service clubs, and similar gatherings. In addition, the state was saturated with "Wanted for Murder" posters similar to that reproduced within Figure 56. Some protests were initially raised against the latter strategy, but many captured ticks have been sent to health departments for laboratory testing.

The medical geography of Rocky Mountain spotted fever in the United States is somewhat unique. It is an example of a disease known to be endemic in one part of a country during one century, and, for some reason not fully understood, suddenly becoming endemic in a different part of a country. Natural ecological settings in the two areas are only partially similar. One striking difference is that tick vectors are different. Whether the changing distributions of Rocky Mountain spotted fever in the United States are actually a clearcut example of relocation

ROCKY MOUNTAIN SPOTTED FEVER

GENERAL INFORMATION

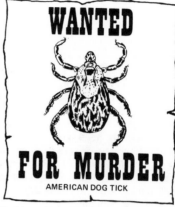

WANTED

FOR MURDER

AMERICAN DOG TICK

In South Carolina, Rocky Mountain Spotted Fever is primarily a disease of women and young children. In 1973, there were 32 cases reported in the state; in 1974, 55 cases were reported, with 5 deaths. Since this year's Rocky Mountain Spotted Fever season is about to begin, the State Department of Health and Environmental Control would like to take this opportunity to acquaint you with the facts about this disease.

The disease is transmitted by the bite of an infected tick. In South Carolina, the tick most often implicated is the American Dog Tick. As its name indicates, this tick is frequently found on dogs. It will also feed readily on humans if they invade its habitat. The places most likely to harbor ticks are those areas with weeds and heavy underbrush. The ticks congregate along paths and wait on vegetation for any animal to pass. If an animal or person brushes against the vegetation, the tick clings to the fur or clothing and searches for a place to feed on the skin. Only about one tick in twenty is infected, and the tick may be attached from 4 to 6 hours before it transmits the disease. If the tick is removed during this time, even an infected tick may not transmit the disease.

THE SYMPTOMS OF ROCKY MOUNTAIN SPOTTED FEVER

The symptoms of Rocky Mountain Spotted Fever may appear from 2 to 12 days after the bite of an infected tick. The symptoms include: sudden chills, high fever, severe headache, and other aches and pains. A distinct rash usually appears on the third day of the disease. The wrists, ankles, and back are the first to show the rash, which may be mistaken for measles.

PRECAUTIONS AGAINST ROCKY MOUNTAIN SPOTTED FEVER

1. Avoid areas with weeds and underbrush when possible.
2. Wear good protective clothing in woods and bushy areas.
3. Use a good tick repellant.
4. Protect your pets by using flea collars or flea/tick repellants.
5. Check children closely at least twice a day for ticks. Look especially behind the ears and on the scalp.
6. If ticks become attached, remove them as soon as possible without breaking off their mouthparts. (Grasp the ticks and pull out firmly, without jerking or twisting.)

In order to determine if a particular tick is infected, ticks removed from persons should be taken alive to your local Health Department or to your family physician. Results of the test will be sent only to physicians and Health Departments.

Live ticks may be transported in a small, clean, tightly capped bottle containing a piece of paper towel moistened with one drop of water. Do not perforate the cap. The following information should be included with the tick: date collected, county, name and address of the person on whom the tick was found, and person who collected the tick. The name and telephone number of the family physician should be included so that he may be notified if the tick is infected. For more information please contact your county health department or the Division of Vector Control, South Carolina Department of Health and Environmental Control.

Fig. 56. This information is an example of the efforts of the South Carolina Department of Health and Environmental Control to educate the general public about risks of Rocky Mountain Spotted Fever within the state.

diffusion may never be truly known. The medical geography of this disease raises general questions about the geographic diffusion of diseases in general discussed in the next chapter.

NOTES

[1] C. Gregory Knight. "The Geography of Vectored Diseases," in John M. Hunter (ed.), *The Geography of Health and Disease.* Chapel Hill: University of North Carolina, Department of Geography (1974), pp. 46–80.

[2] A. G. Voronov. "The Geographical Environment and Human Health," *Soviet Geography,* Vol. 18 (1977), pp. 230–237.

[3] Jacques M. May. "Medical Geography: Its Methods and Objectives," *Geographical Review,* Vol. 40 (1950), pp. 9–41.

[4] Jacques M. May (ed.). *Studies in Disease Ecology.* New York: Hafner (1961).

[5] Wendy H. Waddell, Robert G. Pierleoni, and Emanuel Suter (eds.). *International Health Perspectives: An Introduction in Five Volumes.* New York: Springer (1977).

[6] Denis P. Burkitt. "Geographical Distribution," in D. P. Burkitt and D. H. Wright (eds.), *Burkitt's Lymphoma.* Edinburgh: E. S. S. Livingstone (1970), pp. 186–197.

[7] A. J. Haddow. "Epidemiological Evidence Suggesting an Infective Element in the Aetiology," in D. P. Burkitt and D. H. Wright (eds.), op. cit., pp. 198–209.

[8] N. D. McGlashan. "The African Lymphoma in Central Africa," *International Journal of Cancer,* Vol. 4 (1969), pp. 113–120.

[9] Robert W. Roundy. "Altitudinal Mobility and Disease Hazards for Ethiopian Populations," *Economic Geography,* Vol. 52 (1976), pp. 103–115.

[10] V. A. Yelizarov. "Data on the Medical Geography of Ethiopia," *Izvestiya Vsesoyuznogo Geograficheskogo Obshchestva,* No. 3 (1974), pp. 223–230.

[11] M. Sh. Ishankulov, B. A. Aydarkhanov, and M. Ye. Zel'tser. "Natural Cause-and-Effect Relationships and the Prediction of Endemic Goitre," *Soviet Geography,* Vol. 16 (1975), pp. 169–185.

[12] Joseph B. Schiel, Jr. and Anita Joan Wepfer. "Distributional Aspects of Endemic Goitre in the United States," *Economic Geography,* Vol. 52 (1976), pp. 116–126.

[13] Rais Akhtar. "Goitre in the Kumaon Region of India," *Social Science and Medicine* (Medical Geography), forthcoming (1978).

[14] Robert L. Mitchell. "Trace Elements in Soils and Factors that Affect Their Availability," in Helen L. Cannon and Howard C. Hopps (eds.), *Geochemical Environment in Relation to Health and Disease.* Boulder: The Geological Society of America (1972), pp. 9–16.

[15] Harry V. Warren, Robert E. DeLavault, and Christine H. Cross. "Possible Correlations Between Geology and Some Disease Patterns," *Annals of the New York Academy of Sciences,* Vol. 136 (1967), pp. 657–710.

[16] H. O. Warren. "Medical Geology and Geography," *Science,* Vol. 48 (1965), pp. 534–539.

[17] See Chapter 2, note 8.

[18] R. W. Armstrong. "Medical Geography and Its Geologic Substrate," in Helen L. Cannon and Howard C. Hopps (eds.), *Environmental Geochemistry in Health and Disease.* Boulder: The Geological Society of America (1971), pp. 211–219.

[19] "How Does Geochemical Environment Affect Patterns of Disease?" *News Report,* National Academy of Sciences, July 1976.

[20] Robert Corbett. "Geology and Water Characteristics," unpublished manuscript, Department of Geology, The University of Akron.

[21] A. A. Shoshin. "Geographical Aspects of Public Health," *Soviet Geography,* Vol. 5 (1964), pp. 72–78.

[22] See Chapter 1, note 33.

[23] Ibid.

[24] I. A. Khlebovich and V. I. Chudnova, and L. I. Soboleva. "Medical-Geography Study of the Formation of Population of the Ob' River Region," *Soviet Geography,* Vol. 9 (1968), pp. 106–112.

[25] L. I. Soboleva. "Medical-Geography Aspects of the Design of the Ust'-Ilimsk Industrial Node," *Soviet Geography,* Vol. 15 (1974), pp. 422–428.

[26] V. P. Byakov. "Materials on the Medical Geography of Mountain Landscapes," *Soviet Geography,* Vol. 3 (1962), pp. 20–41.

[27] G. T. Ivanov. "Some Data on the Medical Geography of the European North of the RSFSR," *Soviet Geography,* Vol. 3 (1962), pp. 42–58.

[28] Hiran M. Dutta and Ashok K. Dutt. "Malarial Ecology: A Global Perspective," *Social Science and Medicine (Medical Geography),* Vol. 12 (1978), pp. 69–84.

[29] Charles F. Kovacik. "Health Conditions and Town Growth in Colonial and Antebellum South Carolina," *Social Science and Medicine (Medical Geography),* Vol. 12 (1978), pp. 131–136.

[30] R. Mansell Prothero. *Migrants and Malaria.* London: Longmans (1965).

[31] A. T. A. Learmonth. "Some Contrasts in the Regional Geography of Malaria in India and Pakistan," *Transactions of the Institute of British Geographers,* Vol. 23 (1957), pp. 37–59.

[32] L. Schuyler Fonaroff. "Man and Malaria in Trinidad: Ecological Perspectives of a Changing Health Hazard," *Annals,* Association of American Geographers, Vol. 58 (1968), pp. 526–556.

[33] George MacDonald. *Dynamics of Tropical Disease.* London: Oxford University Press (1973).

[34] M. Farooq. "Historical Development" in N. Ansari (ed.), *Epidemiology and Control of Schistosomiasis (Bilharziasis).* Baltimore: University Park Press (1973), pp. 1–16.

[35] Kenneth C. Haddock. "The Ecology of Schistosomiasis in Puerto Rico," unpublished Master's thesis, Michigan State University (1969).

[36] Willard H. Wright. "Schistosomiasis as a World Problem," *Bulletin, New York Academy of Medicine,* Vol. 44 (1968), pp. 301–312.

[37] Ernest C. Faust, Paul C. Beaver, and Rodney C. Jung. *Animal Agents and Vectors of Human Disease.* 3rd ed. Philadelphia: Lea and Febiger (1968). World Health Organization. "Nature and Extent of the Problem of Bilharziasis," *Chronicle, World Health Organization,* Vol. 13 (1959), p. 2. George W. Hunter, J. Clyde Swartzwelder, and David F. Clyde. *Tropical Medicine.* 5th ed. Philadelphia: W. B. Saunders Co. (1976). Raul A. Marcial-Rojas. "Schistosomiasis Mansoni" in Raul A. Marcial-Rojas (ed.), *Pathology of Protozoal and Helminthic Diseases.* Baltimore: Williams and Wilkins (1971), pp. 373–413.

[38] Emile A. Malek. "The Ecology of Schistosomiasis" in Jacques M. May (ed.), *Studies in Disease Ecology.* New York: Hafner (1961), pp. 261–327.

[39] Frederick F. Ferguson. "The Ecology of Schistosoma in Puerto Rico," *Bulletin, New York Academy of Medicine,* Vol. 44 (1968), pp. 231–244.

[40] George MacDonald, op. cit.

[41] William R. Jobin, Frederick F. Ferguson, and Juan R. Palmer. "Control of Schistosomiasis in Guayama and Arroyo, Puerto Rico," *Bulletin, World Health Organization,* Vol. 42 (1970), pp. 151–156.

[42] Also see Fenwich and T. A. Jorgensen, "The Effect of a Control Programme Against *Schistosoma mansoni* on the Prevalence and Intensity of Infection on an Irrigated Sugar Estate in Northern Tanzania," *Bulletin, World Health Organization,* Vol. 47 (1972), pp. 579–586.

[43] Peter R. Dalton. "A Socioecological Approach to the Control of *Schistosoma mansoni* in St. Lucia," *Bulletin, World Health Organization,* Vol. 54 (1976), pp. 587–595.

[44] G. O. Unrau. "Individual Household Water Supplies as a Control Measure Against *Schistosoma mansoni,*" *Bulletin, World Health Organization,* Vol. 52 (1975), pp. 1–8.

[45] P. Jordan, Lilian Woodstock, G. O. Unrau, and J. A. Cook. "Control of *Schistosoma mansoni* Transmission by Provision of Domestic Water Supplies: A Preliminary Report of a Study in St. Lucia," *Bulletin, World Health Organization,* Vol. 52 (1975), pp. 9–20.

[46] Peter Jordan. "Chemotherapy of Schistosomiasis," *Bulletin, New York Academy of Medicine,* Vol. 44 (1968), pp. 245–258.

[47] See Chapter 3, note 33.

[48] William McD. Hammon and William C. Reeves. "California Encephalitis Virus, A Newly Described Agent, I. Evidence of Natural Infection in Man and Other Animals," *California and Western Medicine,* Vol. 77 (1952), pp. 303–309.

[49] William McD. Hammon, William C. Reeves, and Gladys Sather. "California Encephalitis Virus, A Newly Described Agent, II. Isolations and Attempts to Identify and Characterize the Agent," *Journal of Immunology,* Vol. 69 (1952), pp. 493–510.

[50] Henry G. Cramblett, Howard Stegmiller, and Calvin Spencer. "California Encephalitis Virus Infections in Children," *Journal American Medical Association,* Vol. 198 (1966), pp. 108–112.

[51] Willy Burgdorfer, Verne F. Newhouse, and Leo A. Thomas. "Isolation of California Encephalitis Virus From the Blood of a Snowshoe Hare (*Lepus americanus*) in Western Montana," *American Journal of Hygiene,* Vol. 73 (1961), pp. 344–349. V. Bardos and V. L. Danielova. "The Tahyna Virus–A Virus Isolated From Mosquitoes in Czechoslovakia," *Journal of Hygiene, Epidemiology, Microbiology and Immunology,* Vol. 3 (1959), pp. 264–276.

[52] Frederick A. Murphy and Philip H. Coleman. "California Group Arboviruses: Immuno-diffusion Studies," *Journal of Immunology,* Vol. 99 (1967), pp. 276–284. Wayne H. Thompson and Alfred S. Evans. "California Encephalitis Virus Studies in Wisconsin," American Journal of Epidemiology, Vol. 81 (1965), pp. 230–244.

[53] Richard L. Berry, Margaret A. Parsons, Barbara J. LaLonde et al. "Studies on the Epidemiology of California Encephalitis in an Endemic Area in Ohio in 1971," *The American Journal of Tropical Medicine and Hygiene,* Vol. 24 (1975), pp. 992–998.

[54] N. B. Birulya and L. I. Zalutskaya. "The Geography of Natural Infection Foci of Tick-Borne Encephalitis in the Territory of the USSR," *Izvestiya Akademii Nauk SSSR, Seriya Geograficheskaya,* No. 4 (1967), pp. 32–43.

[55] Pascal James Imperato. *The Treatment and Control of Infectious Diseases in Man.* Springfield: Charles C. Thomas (1974).

[56] R. E. Dyer. "Rocky Mountain Spotted Fever" in Thomas G. Hull (ed.), *Diseases Transmitted from Animals to Man.* 4th ed. Springfield: Charles C. Thomas (1955), pp. 580–590. Franklin H. Top, Sr. and Paul F. Wehrle (eds.). *Communicable and Infectious Diseases.* St. Louis: C. V. Mosby Co. (1972). Guy P. Youmans, Philip Y. Paterson, Herbert M. Sommers. *The Biologic and Clinical Basis of Infectious Diseases.* Philadelphia: W. B. Saunders Co. (1975). Earl L. Atwood, John T. Lamb, and Daniel E. Sonenshine. "The Ecology of Rocky Mountain Spotted Fever in Eastern United States with Particular Reference to Virginia," *Proceedings, Eighth Annual Conference, Southeastern Association of Game and Fish Commissioners* (1964), pp. 1–10. Daniel E. Sonenshine and Carleton M. Clifford.

"Contrasting Incidence of Rocky Mountain Spotted Fever in Ticks Infesting Wild Birds in Eastern U.S. Piedmont and Coastal Areas, with Notes on the Ecology of these Ticks," *Journal of Medical Entomology,* Vol. 10 (1973), pp. 497–502. R. R. Parker, "Rocky Mountain Spotted Fever: Results of Fifteen Years' Prophylactic Vaccination," *American Journal of Tropical Medicine,* Vol. 21 (1941), pp. 369–383.

[57] Earl L. Atwood, John T. Lamb, and Daniel E. Sonenshine. "The Ecology of Rocky Mountain Spotted Fever in Eastern United States with Particular Reference to Virginia," *Proceedings, Eighth Annual Conference, Southeastern Association of Game and Fish Commissions,* October, 1964.

[58] Richard Rothenberg and Daniel E. Sonenshine. "Rocky Mountain Spotted Fever in Virginia: Clinical and Epidemiologic Features," *Journal of Medical Entomology,* Vol. 7 (1970), pp. 663–669.

[59] Daniel E. Sonenshine, Allen H. Peters, and Gerald F. Levy. "Rocky Mountain Spotted Fever in Relation to Vegetation in the Eastern United States, 1951–1971," *American Journal of Epidemiology,* Vol. 96 (1972), pp. 59–69.

[60] J. E. Smadel. "Status of the Rickettsioses in the United States," *Annals of Internal Medicine,* Vol. 51 (1959), pp. 421–435.

[61] Data were supplied by Richard Parker, South Carolina State Epidemiologist, and Michael Loving, Entomologist for the Division of Vector Control.

[62] Land use data were supplied by Professor David Cowen of the University of South Carolina, Department of Geography.

[63] Population forecasts were supplied by Lynn Shirley of the University of South Carolina, Department of Geography.

Chapter 5

STUDIES OF DISEASE DIFFUSION

The term diffusion implies a spreading, or pouring out, from some central source. To explain the spread of disease as diffusion is particularly appropriate in studies of infectious ailments. There are many works available from a variety of sources intended to explain the diffusion of disease within one context or another. The early attempts of August Hirsch in the 19th century represent accounts of mechanisms possibly contributing to the diffusion of disease from a pathogenetic point of view.[1] Such an approach is particularly concerned with the influence of the physical environment; within this context the spread of disease has much common ground with the disease ecological approaches discussed in the previous chapter. An added dimension to environmentally-oriented explanations includes forms of "causal" inference in studies of disease diffusion. Causality is examined in at least two ways in such analyses. One form consists of determination of environmental influences in the spread of disease among human populations and the second implies that human behavior alters environments and contributes to the diffusion of disease. Within the geographical literature studies of disease diffusion take on a fragmented nature in the sense that few, if any, attempts have been made to develop a multifaceted approach to causality. Likewise, a larger literature on the diffusion of disease is even more fragmented. In the course of their work researchers have adopted a variety of approaches and explanations to problems of disease diffusion (see Tables 3 and 4). If these many kinds of studies have any common ground, it rests in the fact that most methodological approaches take on different forms of hypothesis testing intended to offer explanations beyond the generally more static descriptions resulting from

Table 3. Related Approaches to Disease Diffusion

Approach	Historical and general works	Geographic epidemiologies	Public health/ health planning
Type of disease	Vectored and nonvectored infectious.	Vectored and nonvectored infectious.	Infectious (same); Mostly cause of death reporting.
Geographic scale	International; Multiregional or mixed; National; Aspatial.	Scales: general mapping;	General: larger discrete units, e.g., states and counties; Aspatial.
Methods of analysis	Descriptive accounts: "Flows."	Small samples; Selective comparisons; Pathologies/etiology.	Socioeconomic; "Seeding"; Mapping tabular comparisons.
Models	Narrative: replication	Mostly nonparametric.	Descriptions of change regression.
Outcomes/results	*ex post facto,* provision of general information.	Identification of diffusion mechanisms for small samples.	Indicative of change over Time; Costs; Health care provision; Policy indicator.

Table 4. A Comparison of Spatial and Disease Diffusion Approaches

Approach	Literature spatial diffusion	Disease diffusion in Geography
Type of disease	Theoretical basis: broad application to nonvectored infectious diseases.	Nonvectored infectious diseases.
Geographic scale	Variable: generally national to microregional.	Broad range: international to intraurban.
Methods of analysis	Time-series mapping; Mathematical and statistical testing.	"Flow" mapping; Trend surface; Time-distance comparisons.
Models	Broad range of stochastic and deterministic models.	Linear and power models; Planar graphs; Time-Series.
Outcomes/results	Mathematical replication of diffusion processes; Predictive principles.	Retrospective replication of disease diffusion; Predictive: suggestion of barriers.

disease mapping and comparisons with ecological complexes contributing to disease patterns.

General Historical Accounts

When Helmut Jusatz and his colleagues analyzed the diffusion of cerebrospinal meningitis in the *World Atlas of Epidemic Diseases,* they offered an excellent example of the influence of physical environment on the spread of this ailment which passes from human to human over time and space.[2] The comprehensive review of the occurrence and spread of cerebrospinal meningitis developed by August Hirsch now nearly a century ago was offered by Jusatz as detailed background information pertaining to the development of specific knowledge of the pathology of the *meningococcus* causing the problem. According to the earlier literature (prior to World War II), outbreaks of the disease occurred during periods of war and unrest in nations prior to the Industrial Revolution; for example, Napoleonic Europe and the United States during the Civil War. The disease apparently occurs in temporal cycles ranging from four to seven years and was identified by Jusatz as a particular problem in sub-Saharan Africa during the time between the two world wars. Figure 57 shows the diffusion of cerebrospinal meningitis from Ethiopia in 1927 in a westward trend from one oasis to another until its arrival along the Atlantic Coast in Senegal and Guinea in 1941. According to Jusatz, the disease peaked during dry seasons from December to May and was somehow associated with the Harmattan, or hot, dry winds resulting from high pressure to the north. The hypothesis put forth in this analysis thus included climatic influences affecting human behavior over time and space as well as an implied diffusion from east to west along transportation routes. While explanations pertaining to disease diffusion in man and environment can be seen operating in the contribution of Jusatz, emphasis was placed primarily on the effects of environmental conditions and how they influence human behavior and ultimately the diffusion of a nonvectored, infectious disease.

John Hunter's more recent contribution on onchocerciasis in northern Ghana (Sakoti) offers another sort of hypothesis pertaining to the diffusion of disease in an African environment and resultant alterations of human behavior.[3] According to Hunter, the disease may be spread by parasitized black flies. He successfully identified a cycle of advance and retreat of settlement near the Red Volta River and hypothesized that retreat from the riverine areas was due to the spread of river blindness over time. Furthermore, during less severe seasons there were attempts to move settlements closer to the river. During periods when the disease was on the upswing, settlements slowly moved away from the immediate riverine site. Hunter offers an example of how human behavior is modified in relation to cycles of the diffusion of a vectored disease, particularly in areas of more primitive living conditions. (see Figure 58 supporting Hunter's hypothesis). Living conditions relative to levels of economic development also tend to be underlying themes in many historical and general works pertaining to disease diffusion.

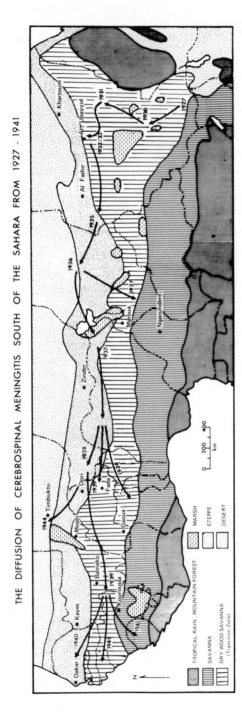

THE DIFFUSION OF CEREBROSPINAL MENINGITIS SOUTH OF THE SAHARA FROM 1927 - 1941

Fig. 57. The westward diffusion of Cerebrospinal Meningitis in Africa south of the Sahara prior to the Second World War (adapted from Rodenwaldt and Jusatz).

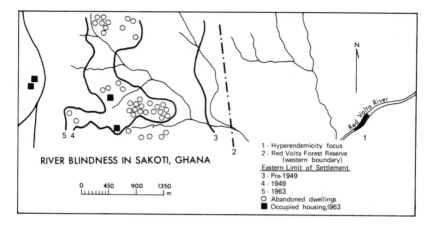

Fig. 58. John Hunter's explanation of the retreat of settlement due to risk of River Blindness.

Historical reconstructions of epidemics of vectored and nonvectored diseases rely on archival research explaining different societies at points in time. Sometimes included are accounts of political conditions which may have indirectly contributed to the spread of disease. One of the most widely studied sagas of the diffusion of disease is the Black Death, or Bubonic plague, in Europe during the middle of the fourteenth century. According to Melvyn Howe, Bubonic plague during those times was primarily a disease of the poor.[4] The pathogen, the *bacillis Pasteurella pestis,* can produce the infection in rats, and fleas from the infected rats in turn transfer the disease to humans. According to most accounts, the Black Death spread into Europe from either Asia or Asia Minor in late 1347.[5] Over a period of the next several years it diffused northward along the Italian Peninsula into France and subsequently Great Britain and Scandinavia (see Figure 59). Densely settled areas were particularly affected; apparently the poor the most severely. It was not uncommon for people living in crowed conditions or small dwellings to sleep on straw which attracted the infected fleas. The presence of domestic animals within homes also contributed greatly to the problem. In fact, according to Banks, it was much later in history before people realized that this combination of factors was responsible for the Black Death as well as other diseases. Improved sanitary conditions in the 19th century ultimately led to decreases in the spread of various vectored diseases.

The spread of black plague through medieval Europe caused millions of deaths. In some instances from 25 to 40% of village populations were lost. The social and economic consequences of the disaster were felt in Europe for centuries. For example, given a decline which may have been as much as a third of the population, agricultural production diminished, areas of cultivated land

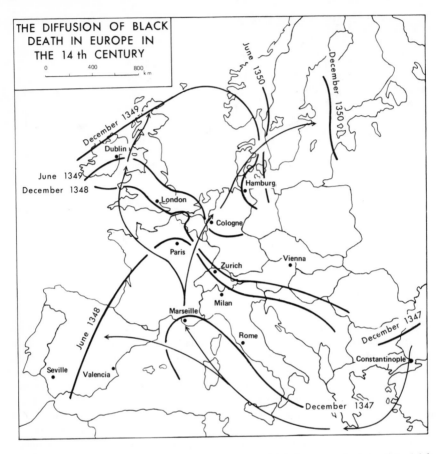

Fig. 59. Diffusion of Bubonic Plague within Europe during the 14th century (after Ziegler, Cartwright, and Howe).

shrank and an overall decrease in wealth resulted. Because the peasant population was greatly affected by the disease, in some locations labor was at a premium and pressures could be put forth on landholders to increase the benefits for laborers.

As the plague swept through Europe, settlements were disrupted in its wake and the result was often migrations of large groups. Given the beliefs of most Europeans at the time, it was not surprising to find religious explanations to the Black Death. In many instances when no solace was found, and death of friends or relatives resulted, the position of the church was substantially weakened.

Concurrently, it was also not surprising to find persecution of Jews, the ultimate European scapegoats historically.

The reconstruction of cholera epidemics is another example of the utility of historical analysis in understanding the diffusion of disease. Man is the prime reservoir for cholera. The several cholera vibrios which spread from one person to another are carried initially by human feces which contaminate water.[6] Environmental conditions favoring the spread of the disease include warm temperatures and prolonged dry spells. The vibrios have a chance to flourish in warm alkaline mediums, and as epidemics diffuse, such secondary sources as food and perhaps even flies can carry the disease. Stages of cholera in humans are characterized by diarrhea followed by copious evacuations, sometimes collapse, and uremia. In a full-blown epidemic or pandemic it is quite possible for humans to contract the disease in more latter stages, and it can be fatal.

The occurrence of cholera is rooted in sub-Asian antiquity. One principal endemic area of cholera has been the delta of the Ganges and Brahmaputra Rivers in Eastern India and Bangladesh. Rodenwalt's account of the cholera epidemic in the mid-1860s is a demonstration of how rapidly a pandemic of the disease can spread throughout the world (see Figure 60).[7] According to Rodenwalt's reconstruction in the *World Atlas of Epidemic Diseases*, cholera spread from its endemic area westward across India and into Africa during 1863 and 1864. At the same time the disease diffused southward through the Malay Peninsula and into the East Indies by 1865. Another track was into China. During the period 1865 to 1867 the disease spread into Europe and Russia, as well as down the West African Coast. By 1866, the pandemic also had reached the New World. While entry into South America is not well known, Rodenwalt's reconstruction suggests that the disease spread up the Rio de La Plata and into the interior of the southern part of South America. Cholera spread rapidly to the Antilles in 1865 and reached Canada and the United States by 1866.

Given the status of sanitary conditions throughout the world in spite of increased standards of living and economic development in more advanced nations, it was not surprising to find the cholera epidemic following water-borne transportation routes initially. Quarantine procedures were initiated in many seaports. Later in the 19th century in conjunction with a general public health movement in more advanced nations, some control measures were developed to counteract the threat of new invasions of cholera. The disease spread in different ways in the United States during the 19th century.[8] Earlier cholera epidemics can definitely be traced to water-borne transportation routes connecting settlement patterns; however, the diffusion of the mid-1860s may have been more a function of the growing hierarchical nature of the urban system in the United States (see Figure 61). This is one example of initial effects of environment on the diffusion of disease in man, followed by man's alteration of the environment.

In *Diseases That Plague Modern Man*, Richard Gallagher explains the utility of the study of the history of communicable disease in understanding modern-day health problems.[9] He describes the study of infectious diseases historically as one of "man's longest interrupted wars." Gallagher also explains how some "new" diseases may not be so new at all, and that as our knowledge of particular

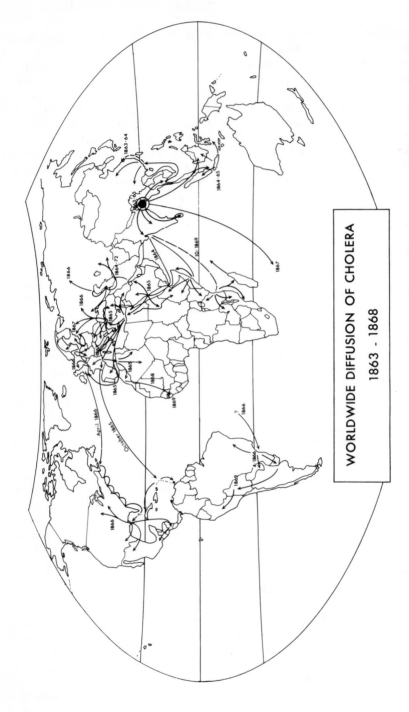

WORLDWIDE DIFFUSION OF CHOLERA

1863 - 1868

Fig. 60. Worldwide diffusion of Cholera from 1863 to 1868 (adapted from Rodenwaldt and Jusatz).

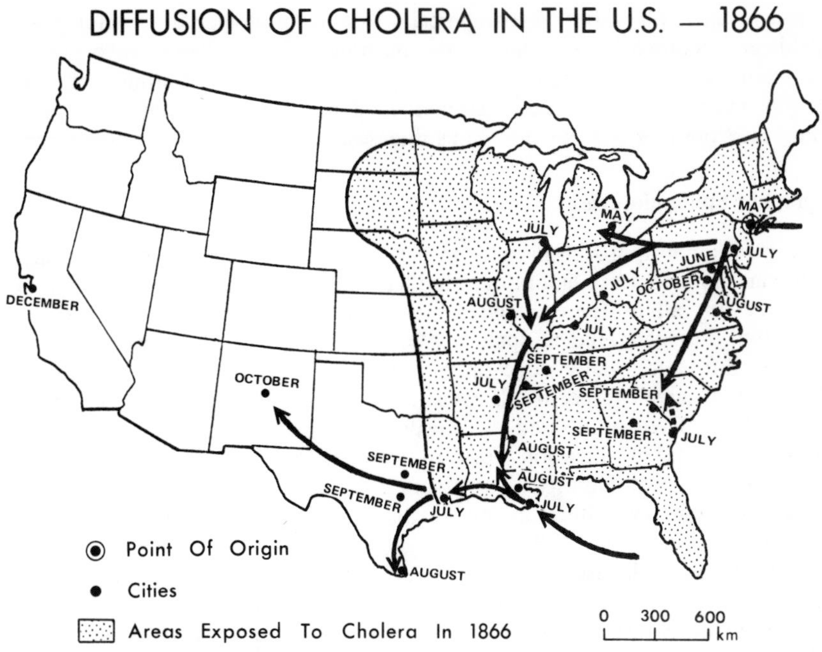

DIFFUSION OF CHOLERA IN THE U.S. — 1866

Fig. 61. Diffusion of Cholera in the United States in 1866.

etiologies increases we can better contain some of these problems. Gallagher offers excellent examples of background which help explain the diffusion and persistence of cholera, influenza, leprosy, malaria, schistosomiasis, onchocerciasis, plague, smallpox, syphilis, and tuberculosis. Developing an understanding of the historical progression of diseases which have a tendency to diffuse in time and space is an integral part of understanding mechanisms contributing to the spread of disease diffusion now.

However, it is too much to assume that the widespread and partially coordinated efforts of the World Health Organization can indeed prevent the diffusion of epidemics of certain communicable diseases throughout developing parts of the world. Indeed, there is a conceptual problem which must be overcome before more fully coordinated efforts of disease control can be implemented. The problem stems from a gap in scale of analysis. Much has been done in the laboratory and a considerable amount of effort can be seen in the works of epidemiologists studying microscale associations of the spread of diseases. At the other extreme, international descriptions of the spread of disease from one country to another in time offer advance warning of pending epidemics. The gap consists of several levels of geographical analysis which must be brought into play. Both geographical and epidemiological methodologies are available to accomplish this. One of the purposes of this chapter is to put forth some examples of different levels of analysis to the end that studies of disease diffusion might be substantially strengthened and, in fact, contribute to controlling the "pouring out" of infectious diseases.

Geographic Epidemiologies

The traditional approach in epidemiological studies involving time and space is to compare and contrast laboratory findings with microscale field investigations. Many, but not all of these analyses rely on relatively small statistical samples. Quite often in such studies spatial interaction of humans is taken into consideration, but it is usually done on a limited basis after interviewing confirmed and suspected cases of specific diseases. Such notions as "seeding" or "sporadic outbreaks" are frequently used as a way of explaining away the possibility of continuous forms of diffusion outward from endemic areas. Still, geographers have as much, if not more, to learn from epidemiologists as the latter do from the general geographic literature on spatial diffusion (discussed subsequently in this chapter).

Many infectious diseases occur in either time series cycles or in nearly normal distributions. For example, Figure 62, based on a report from the Center for Disease Control, shows a comparison of distributions of hepatitis A outbreaks in Portland, Oregon and Buffalo, New York in 1975 and in 1976.[10] By contrast, Figure 63 shows different cycles or "generations" of an epidemic of measles in Akron, Ohio during 1971. Note that with the Portland and Buffalo hepatitis A examples an index case was identified in each instance. Often, as was the case with the Akron measles information, the identification of an index case is not always possible. Of more importance than the actual identification of the index case is the fact that all too often there is a time lag between the realization that a possible epidemic of a disease is taking place and increased reporting. As shown within Figure 62, control measures in the Portland area contributed to a rather rapid decline in what might have been a more normal distribution of hepatitis. In Buffalo the outbreak was spread out over a longer period of time. While often in epidemiological studies such distributions are reconstructed and index cases identified, not enough attention is given to the possibility of diffusion over space as well as time.

In most instances, the purpose of microscale epidemiologic studies of spatial diffusion is to test various hypotheses which have been put forth pertaining to the variable spread of disease-causing agents. Such an example is offered in the works of Wehrle and his colleagues in an analysis of smallpox in a German hospital.[11] Their hypothesis was essentially that within a particular hospital it is possible for smallpox to spread in an airborne fashion. In a classical fashion an index case was identified. This is followed by a time gap presumed to be an infectious period. The distribution of subsequent cases was then shown over time. Wehrle and his colleagues supported their explanation of airborne spread of smallpox within the hospital by making use of the architectural plan of the

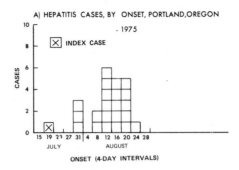

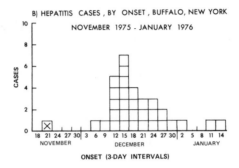

Fig. 62. Distributions of Hepatitis reporting in Portland, Oregon, and Buffalo, New York. Note the identification of index cases in both locations.

structure. It was concluded that the hospital outbreak was unusual because after the index case there was apparently no face-to-face contact among other victims. While Wehrle and his colleagues also attempted to place the outbreak within a larger context of importation of smallpox into Europe over a period from 1960 to 1970, no attempt was made to show spatial relationships. It was not possible to accomplish this because additional information pertaining to sources of origin and method of probable transportation of index cases, while tabulated, was not analyzed within a broader geographic context. Since most of the index cases identified traveled into specific countries initially by air transportation, the overall pattern suggested indicates that sporadic outbreaks are primarily due to the introduction of smallpox exclusively from extraneous geographic sources.

In 1978 the World Health Organization announced that smallpox has been eradicated internationally, but knowledge of the diffusion of past epidemics can help understand many other disease problems.

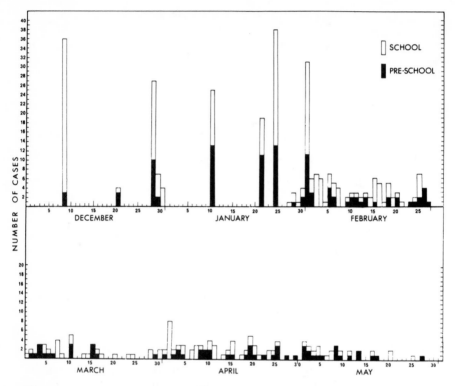

Fig. 63. Cycles of "generations" of measles reporting in Akron, Ohio during an epidemic in the early 1970s.

In testing the airborne diffusion hypothesis in smallpox infections (and classroom contamination), Klauber and Angulo in an analysis of *Variola minor* in Braganca, Paulista County, Brazil, brought me to the conclusion that while there was a possibility of airborne diffusion via droplets of infected dust, they could find no strong evidence that smallpox was spread among students within a classroom due to contamination of desks and materials used ʋy the students.[12] They further hypothesized that the disease may have diffused through direct contacts while students were queuing for classrooms. In a further analysis of the same information, Angulo, Haggett and Pederneiras examined the diffusion of *Variola minor* within a settled area.[13] Using polynomial trend surface analysis, they came to the general conclusion that an endemic center could be located within Braganca Paulista City near the central part of the settlement, and the diffusion of the disease could be traced outward in several directions over time. The study by Angulo, Haggett, and their colleagues is an unusual example wherein an epidemiologist and a geographer knowledgeable in methods of time-space diffusion cooperated in the spatial analysis of microscale disease diffusion. The results showed statistical significance and lent support to the idea that certain infectious diseases can diffuse outward from areas of "sporadic outbreak."

Works explaining the diffusion of infectious diseases from one geographic place to another are not absent from the epidemiological literature. It is more common, however, to find limited use of some of the methods available in spatial analytic research in developing an understanding of the mechanisms contributing to the diffusion of disease. For example, in an analysis of the epidemiology of measles in the U.S. Trust Territory of the Pacific islands, Gould, Herrman, and Witte adhered to the notion of sporadic outbreaks of measles while at the same time offered some indication of how measles diffused from one year to the next among these islands.[14] As is possible with measles infection information, the authors of this work were able to show the cyclical nature of outbreaks by municipalities. Although a study in diffusion, one of the objects of this work was to mathematically examine the time intervals between outbreaks of measles. A generalized negative exponential function was also used to show a distance decay relationship as the epidemic extended from one point in time to another. While a small number of observations was used, the actual observed intervals for several of the districts did approximate the hypothesized or predicted intervals.

In a 1971 contribution to the *British Medical Bulletin* intended to explain epidemics of rare diseases, E. G. Knox offers a review of some time–space studies accomplished by epidemiologists.[15] Knox points out how epidemiology is concerned primarily with knowledge of etiologies (perhaps as opposed to pathogenesis) intended to explain how infections spread from one person to another. Knox indicates how the concept of spread of disease must include the examination of certain spatial elements. In order to accomplish this, according to Knox, it is important to understand the frequency of disease in terms of time intervals and such concepts as overlapping cycles of disease in time and space. He indicates how many of the tests used for nonrandomness can be replaced with either Poisson distributions or negative exponential associations. In many respects he takes to task the common notion in the medical profession and epidemiology that so many diseases are distributed randomly there is simply no point in examining spatial processes. Knox espouses notions of disease mapping within a time series context and indicates examples in the medical literature which use concepts common to geographical diffusion, including network analysis. The techniques Knox disucsses are still essentially microgeographic, and there is some indication in this contribution that studies of time–space associations cannot be accomplished on a national basis.

Public Health and Health Care Planning

In addition to contributions in the historical, epidemiological and medical literature, some studies in health planning and public health examine changes in disease patterns over time and space. The latter approaches are summarized within the context of disease type, geographic scale, models and methods of analysis, and outcomes within Table 3. For example, many of the historical and general works have examined both vectored (plague) and nonvectored infectious diseases. In general, the geographical scale utilized is either international, national, or macroregional. In some instances, no specific geographic scale is utilized. Methods of analysis generally include descriptive accounts and narratives explaining how various diseases diffuse spatially. The narrative accounts are largely replications of past epidemics and offer frameworks for further investigation using archival research. The outcomes provide general information about the historical spread of disease and tend to suggest that such research methods can be particularly fruitful if outbreaks of particular kinds of diseases occur. During the latter part of the 20th century this is particularly possible in both developing nations and countries undergoing various forms of social and political unrest.

Most of the medical-epidemiological studies also concentrate on infectious diseases, both vectored and nonvectored. They depart from the general and historical works in several ways. One major difference is that while much has been written, quite often there is either no attempt to map and statistically test the diffusion of diseases nor are specific spatial examples offered. Furthermore, any mapping included is fairly elementary in nature.

Approaches to disease diffusion in public health rely primarily on biomedical techniques of analysis. As shown within Table 3, much less has been accomplished in examination of disease diffusion mechanisms, particularly in health planning practice. There is substantial reliance on the epidemiological literature, and some time series analyses have been done for some infectious diseases. However, health planning relies more heavily on generalized mapping of mortality data, sometimes indicating changes from one point in time to another. In terms of geographic scale, change mapping has been accomplished primarily with larger discrete units, for example, states and counties. Methods of analysis include general comparisons of national or state data with local health problems and extensive tabulations. There are some examples of "seeding" of infectious diseases offered, but little empirical work has been accomplished in the area of disease diffusion. Models used in such studies describing change rely heavily on regression analysis. Quite often models developed may show general changes in time statistically associated with socioeconomic indicators, but in many instances attempts are made to "explain away" results of regressions by bringing general environmental factors into play. Outcomes generally show macrolevel indicators of change which are in turn often compared to costs of health care and general health care provision. In many instances information from these generalized studies is used in public health in attempts to locate centers of disease prevention. Much more specific analyses need to be brought into play if workers in the health area are to develop the abilities to implement disease control and prevention programs via a disease diffusion framework.

The contributions of some of the methods of analysis and models in the area of medical geography have much to offer in terms of disease control and prevention. One major obstacle appears to be the development of a comprehensive understanding of many of the approaches not considered a part of the geographical literature as well as a synthesis of principles of spatial diffusion with the major approaches mentioned above.

GENERAL GEOGRAPHIC PRINCIPLES OF SPATIAL DIFFUSION

Torsten Hagerstrand's early work on "the propagation of innovation waves" continues to be the basis for many general aspects of spatial diffusion. Some of Hagerstrand's work showed how automobile ownership diffused throughout the province of Skane in Sweden during the 1920s. Hagerstrand's pioneer efforts and other studies have led to a body of geographical knowledge about spatial diffusion. In "Aspects of the Spatial Structure of Social Communication and the Diffusion of Information," also by Hagerstrand, methods of predicting time-space courses or paths of diffusion were explained.[16] In this instance he wrote about "S-shaped" or logistic curves and how such growth curves could be used to explain normal processes of diffusion. Working with probabilities, he explained how the actual diffusion of information and innovations over space could be first replicated within a general information field and then simulated. The example used was the diffusion of rotary clubs in Europe during the 1920s, 1930s, 1940s, and 1950s.[17] It was possible through such a method to measure sequences of growth. Utilizing a methodology based on Hagerstrand's hypothesis, Morrill was able to replicate the spread of Seattle's black ghetto from 1940 to 1960.[18] Based on probabilities developed from past knowledge and utilization of the mean information field and simulation modeling, Morrill was further able to simulate and forecast ghetto expansion within Seattle.

By the late 1960s, our knowledge of the diffusion process had grown. When Gould synthesized this literature in 1969, he explained how the processes of spatial diffusion represent an understanding of the meshing of time and space.[19] Drawing form the works of Brown and Moore, Gould explained four critically important types of diffusion.[20] One process is known as expansion diffusion. Within this general context communications and ideas spread spatially and temporally until increasing numbers of individuals become aware of phenomena. Another important kind of diffusion is known as relocation diffusion; the most common example is migration, or complete relocation, from one geographical area to another. The probable relocation of Rocky Mountain spotted fever mentioned in Chapter 4 is such a case. Yet another process, quite common to medical studies, consists of contagious diffusion wherein one infected individual might contaminate several others who, in turn, spread a disease to many more individuals. Without controls, contagious diffusion of disease can be geometrical in progression. Indications of the spread of such infectious diseases can be seen in the general and historical works mentioned within this chapter. The fourth important type of spreading out, sometimes in a leap-frogging fashion, consists of hierarchical diffusion. Within this context, ideas, innovations and, in fact, contagious diseases can spread from a larger urban center to next larger settlements in accordance with a hierarchy of size. This is particularly the case within well developed urban systems.

In general, many of these types of diffusion can be summarized as waves of diffusion strength with distance away from source areas. In addition to the identification of regularities in the process of spatial diffusion, it is also possible to identify different kinds of barriers. The most common barriers consist of various physiographic features. Equally important barriers to the diffusion process consist of political boundaries. In some instances linguistic barriers can inhibit the process of diffusion. With the process of disease diffusion, different kinds of control programs in different political units may serve as barriers.

The general process of diffusion over space can be summarized mathematically (see Table 4). For example, many kinds of spatial diffusion can be identified as taking place within a normal distribution beginning with innovators and moving to an early majority followed by a late majority and laggards. Disease distributions can be translated into the well-known S-shaped or logistic curve identified by the following formulation (see Figure 64):

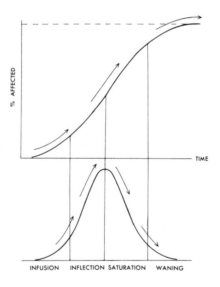

Fig. 64. An adaptation of spatial diffusion phases to disease diffusion. The first quartile is considered the infusion stage, the second, inflection, the third, saturation, and the fourth, waning.

1. Infusion through the 25th percentile
2. Inflection to the 50th percentile
3. Saturation through the 75th percentile
4. Waning to the upper limits.

As the cumulative portion of victims increases such stages can be determined. This has been expressed both in terms of quartiles and quintiles of a distribution, and depending upon the rate of spread, different breaks in the cumulative distribution become identifiable stages.

As earlier indicated by Hagerstrand (1952), processes of spatial diffusion operate at a variety of geographic scales.[21] Such an approach is particularly important to understanding the diffusion of disease and represents one mechanism whereby the gap between micro and macroscale levels of analysis might be closed. Variable levels of understanding geographic scale were explained in 1968 by Stafford Beer as "cones of resolution."[22] Examination of Figure 65 reveals how such layering of diffusion might be meaningful to medical geography. The general context of national, regional, and local planes of diffusion is also discussed by Meyer, Semple, and Brown in their explanations of cones of resolution within a context of different types of diffusion processes.[23] Semple and Brown clarify the question of spatial diffusion from both a functional and spatial perspective and offer a further summary of the literature on spatial diffusion. Again, aspects of variable geographic scale are brought into play. Meyer further explains how micro and macroscale levels of analysis can be viewed from a variety of approaches and offers four dimensions, including spatial scale, diffusion as opposed to adoption activity, type of adoption and types of decision making.

One aspect of particular importance within this body of knowledge consists of diffusion within and among national urban systems. Berry's contribution of the diffusion of urban systems themselves and how they have grown emphasizes this point, and such notions can be of utility in studies of spatial diffusion over time.[24] In a 1970 publication, Pedersen examined innovation diffusion in a national urban system using Chile as a case in point. Pedersen identified a multiplicity of diffusion processes over time in Latin America and explained how such an approach can be used in planning economic development.[25] In an analysis of the diffusion of black and white television within the United States, Berry was able to show how the process operated from the 1930s through the 1950s.[26] Those parts of the United States first licensing television stations were in the more urban industrialized northeastern part of the country. Gradually, over time, particularly after World War II, the availability of television reception diffused outward from that core area. Both empirical and conceptual studies in spatial diffusion processes can be found in two special issues (1974 and 1975) of *Economic Geography* edited by Brown.[27]

In a summary of diffusion models, Haggett explained how various stages, including a first or primary stage, a second or diffusion stage, a third or condensing stage, and a fourth or saturation stage can be identified spatially and mathematically.[28] Haggett used some principles developed by Bailey and was one

LAYERS OF DIFFUSION

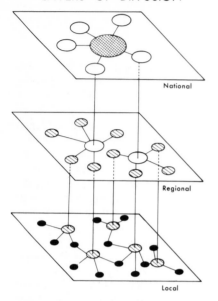

Fig. 65. The well-known presentation of layers of diffusion at different geographic scales.

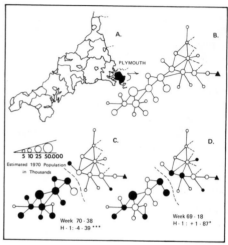

Fig. 66. Peter Haggett's analysis of the diffusion of measles.

of the first geographers to "bridge the gap" and show how the study of spatial diffusion can be used in understanding the spread of disease. Haggett further demonstrated how a contagious process could be represented on a planar graph utilizing some principles of network theory. The various diagrammatical representations shown within Figure 66 explain how contagious regions can be graphically depicted utilizing epidemiological data.[29] The utilization of some general theories of spatial diffusion as outlined by geographers, upon occasion drawing from epidemiological models, is a necessary ingredient in enhancing epidemiological studies particularly devoid of an understanding of geographic scale.

Geographic Contributions to the Analysis of Disease Diffusion

While some geographic studies of disease diffusion have already been mentioned, discussion of several additional contributions assists in understanding viable research methodologies. Table 4 shows broad categories of analysis. Depending upon the type of disease studies, the spatial diffusion literature offers a general theoretical basis, although not exclusively with respect to understanding nonvectored infectious diseases.

However, most successful analyses of this kind are concerned with such communicable diseases. A broad range of such studies has been accomplished at different scales. Methods of analysis include time series mapping and the mathematical and statistical testing. Within some studies such techniques as trend surface analysis and related statistical comparisons have been accomplished. An equally broad range of stochastic and deterministic models result from the general diffusion literature, and geographers have identified such aspects of disease diffusion as negative exponential distance decay functions, cumulative distributions, planar graphs and time series studies. Outcomes include mathematical replications of disease diffusion processes as well as certain principles which can be used to predict the spread of epidemics. Given such knowledge, it is possible to offer suggestions for such preventive measures as the erection of barriers in attempts to limit the spatial diffusion of diseases.

At the state level, Florin has offered an analysis of the general diffusion of mortality within Massachusetts from 1750 to 1850.[30] Utilizing trend surface analysis, Florin was able to explain how the diffusion of increasing average age of death diffused outward from the coastal areas of settlement prior to the American Revolution to western Massachusetts by 1850. In addition, he was able to distinguish microregional urban to suburban diffusion patterns during the later stages within overall parts of the New England region. Use of trend surface analysis to explain mortality spread proves to be highly successful in studies of spatial diffusion (reference is again made to the study of smallpox diffusion within Braganca Paulista).

Also utilizing a trend surface methodology with accompanying analysis of variance statistics, Kwofie studied the spatial and temporal diffusion of cholera in West Africa during the early 1970s.[31] The particular disease problem analyzed by Kwofie was actually part of a major ten-year diffusion pattern of cholera outward from endemic areas (see Figure 67). Kwofie identified the spread of cholera in West Africa in more detail by segmenting the epidemic spread into three phases: primary saturation; saturation, and saturation waning. Figure 68 shows directions of the spread. During the primary saturation phase, for example, the epidemic generally spread from west to east. A quadratic surface best fits this primary phase. During a second, or saturation phase in 1971, a cubic surface explained how the epidemic changed its direction from a general west to east trend and recirculated to the West African coast as well as to the interior. At the same time, there were indications of some movement from the central sub-Saharan area toward the west. By the time the waning phase developed, general trends could be identified (a cubic surface) continuing from west to east as well as east to west, centralizing in the Sahelian countries. While Kwofie's study indicates a pressing need for more treatment facilities, it also poses the question of endemicity of cholera within Africa.

In a more detailed and comprehensive analysis, Stock also examined cholera in Africa within an overall spatial diffusion framework.[32] Stock identified four types of cholera diffusion within various parts of Africa. These included coastal,

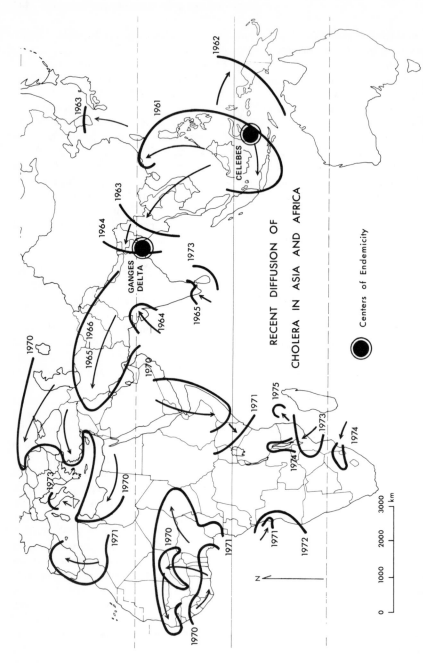

Fig. 67. The recent diffusion of Cholera in Asia and Africa (after Stock and the World Health Organization).

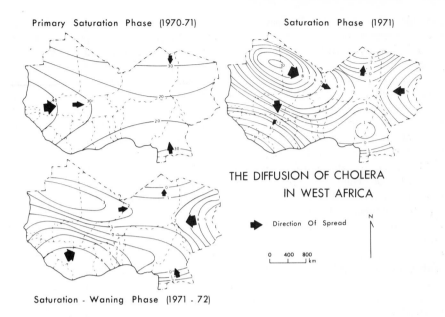

Primary Saturation Phase (1970-71)   Saturation Phase (1971)

THE DIFFUSION OF CHOLERA
IN WEST AFRICA

Direction Of Spread

0   400   800
|____|____| km

Saturation - Waning Phase (1971 - 72)

Fig. 68. Kwofie's version of the diffusion of Cholera in Western Africa showing primary saturation, saturation, and saturation waning. Kwofie developed these maps as polynomial trend surfaces.

riverine, urban hierarchical, and radial contact diffusion. Stock first indicated cholera reporting areas in Africa from 1970 to 1975. These included parts of the horn of Africa (Ethiopia, Kenya, and Somalia), Mozambique, Angola, and large sections of West Africa already identified by Kwofie. In the hard hit West Africa area, for example, Stock accomplished a detailed analysis of diffusion of cholera by identifying coastal diffusion routes, riverine routes, urban hierarchical routes, and more localized areas of radial contact. The diffusion of cholera in East Africa's horn was found to be more linear in nature, starting in the Red Sea-Yemen area and gradually moving southward into Somalia and Kenya. However, localized areas of contact diffusion could be identified. In Angola and Mozambique the epidemic generally followed routes of transportation with localized outbreaks.

Stock developed specific models of cholera spread, interfacing with general notions of diffusion. His model of coastal diffusion, for example, showed a first phase where the disease spread among coastal fishing villages. Cholera then progressed to larger coastal urban centers and spread into the interior, both along transportation lines and (at times) in relation to city size. Stock also showed how riverine linear contact diffusion took place, particularly in the middle Niger Valley. Also within the general context of diffusion theory, Stock offered certain examples of permeable and impermeable barriers, and the possibility of epidemics being channeled in certain directions to later expand into susceptible areas. In general, Stock's contribution is one of the more comprehensive analyses linking disease etiology with general principles of spatial diffusion. Following this approach, a disease is examined first internationally, generally examining spread from one country to another. It then is possible to identify layers of diffusion within regions and local areas. It can also be demonstrated how several different kinds of diffusion operate either simultaneously or from one phase to another of an epidemic. As already mentioned, such knowledge is useful in planning for the prevention of the spatial diffusion of many disease forms.

Studies of the spread of hepatitis are another example of meshing principles of spatial diffusion with the geographic epidemiology of infectious diseases. Brownlea demonstrated the utility of this method in an analysis of infectious hepatitis incidence in the Wollongong settlement system between 1954 to 1970.[33] Brownlea initially found that as the settlement system spread outward from growth centers, environmental conditions in new growth areas lead to specific sanitation problems. He identified infectious hepatitis "vectors" in relation to food and water supplies. A general linear pattern of hepatitis which spread along certain routes, particularly in areas of recent growth, could be identified. Brownlea noted certain ecological "pathways" moving into and progressing along what he termed "clinical fronts." He proved mathematically that infectious hepatitis was moving at a rate faster than random. Actual and predicted locations of moving fronts were compared and a definite association with outer suburbs and similar areas undergoing change was made. Within a general model building and testing context, several principles of diffusion of disease were examined by Brownlea. In an initial step, for example, Brownlea estimated the actual input of susceptibles probably exposed to the virus. In many but not all instances he identified diffusion using a general logistic curve. When that was not possible, a general linear curve showing increases of mixing in the population over time and with the number of contacts was used. In another phase, Brownlea identified actual "ecological pathways" by pinpointing places of origin and subsequently monitoring movements. By further utilizing simulation procedures as put forth by Hagerstrand, Brownlea was able to use general field theory in an attempt to forecast various kinds of diffusion of infectious hepatitis. He found a general distance decay function operating along the identified clinical front. In a fashion similar to Stock, several factors, including growth and settlement size, needed to be considered.

In a more recent examination of the spread of viral hepatitis in Tasmania, McGlashan used the municipal network as a basis for temporal comparisons.[34] He also identified a distance decay association operating outward from endemic centers. In contrast with Brownlea's earlier findings, however, McGlashan examined "discrete hepatitis regions" or subsystems within Tasmania. He showed how the disease diffused outward in a more or less radial-hierarchical fashion, only to decrease in reporting after reaching a certain distance away from the endemic centers. McGlashan pointed out how hepatitis-A is still a significant public health problem in Tasmania, and his identification of general subsystems of outward endemic diffusion are examples of the methodology geographers have to offer the public health sector toward overall disease prevention.

Another disease requiring this kind of analysis is influenza. When Hunter and Young examined the diffusion of influenza in England and Wales in a 1971 study, they found certain common ground with other workers in the area of disease diffusion.[35] One of the hypothesized associations they tested on a national basis was that the diffusion of influenza outward from possibly endemic centers in Britain to the surrounding countryside was related to population potential. By testing against population potential, they found that this measure had some influence at the onset of the 1957 epidemic (see Figure 69). After the initial epidemic wave, there appeared to be certain "virus flowlines" emanating outward from various population centers at a microlevel. Such findings are somewhat similar to those of McGlashan in his study of hepatitis-A in Tasmania and also parallel the findings of Stock at the microregional level. This possibility of radial contact diffusion during successive waves of an epidemic is of particular importance to studies of disease diffusion. Likewise, given the current problem of constantly changing or "drifting" strains of influenza, general principles of spatial diffusion can be utilized in attempting to develop a better understanding of the spread of influenza in space and time.

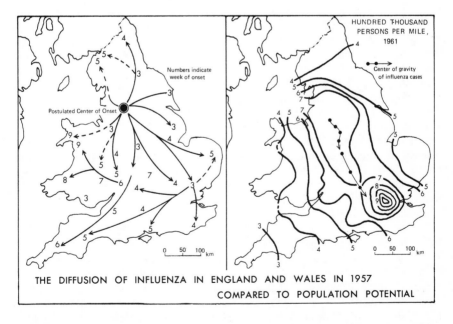

THE DIFFUSION OF INFLUENZA IN ENGLAND AND WALES IN 1957 COMPARED TO POPULATION POTENTIAL

Fig. 69. The diffusion of Influenza in England and Wales in 1957 compared to population potential (after Hunter and Young).

THE PROBLEM OF INFLUENZA DIFFUSION:
A CASE STUDY

The term influenza comes from Italian and simply means "influence."[36] Different historical accounts indicate that the ailment was so named because of perceived influences of either cold weather, the cold wind, or even the stars. The disease has an incubation period of from two to seven days, followed by the sudden onset of headache, nausea, chills or fever, and human temperatures rising to 39°C.[37] Many symptoms are similar to a "common cold" and aching muscles are sometimes manifested in this disease that normally lasts from three to six days. It is primarily a respiratory ailment affecting cells in the lining of the nose, throat, trachea, and lungs. At this time there is no known effective treatment for influenza. Mass innoculation has limited long-term results in terms of disease prevention. Part of the problem is that there are actually several types of influenza virus (A, B, and C).[38] In addition there are hundreds of different strains or subgroups within the three main types. There are periodic shifts and/or drifts in various strains (explained below). In terms of medical geography, influenza is ubiquitous globally. In addition, the disease has a history of regular epidemics occurring from every two to three years, and major pandemics diffusing throughout the world on the average of about every two and a half decades.

Gallagher's accounts of the history of influenza explain how the disease was known in Rome in the 2nd century B.C. Outbreaks severe enough to create extremely excessive mortality show up periodically in European history. For example, the disease in severe form diffused through Europe in the late 12th century. It showed up again in major proportions in the 15th century. Beveridge developed a reconstruction of major and minor influenza pandemics from approximately 1729.[39] Figure 70, adapted from the work of Beveridge, gives some indication of major and minor pandemics. Normal epidemic cycles are not included within this illustration. The most severe pandemics are known to have occurred in 1732-33, 1781-82, 1847-48, 1889-90 (known as the Asiatic or "Russian" flu), 1918 (the most severe: "Spanish" influenza). 1957 and 1968. Some studies on influenza suggest that the world can now expect a pandemic of infuenza in some proportion approximately every decade. However, within this century the two most severe epidemics occurred in 1918 and 1957. While there is still no "cure" for influenza, much is now known about the nature of the disease, particularly the relationship between antigenic shift and the diffusion of influenza.

Our knowledge of the influenza virus dates to the early 1930s. In the late 1920s, Richard Shope experimented with animals and offered the first proof that there is a definite association between influenza in humans and in different kinds of animals, particularly pigs, horses, and perhaps some fowl.[40] Shope isolated the influenza virus and published that information in 1931. In 1933, further research in the identification of influenza virus was successfully accomplished by Christopher Andrewes and Wilson Smith working in London. Subsequent findings have led to the identification of the major A type virus which attacks adults, the less ubiquitous but occasionally more harmful B type virus and the even less

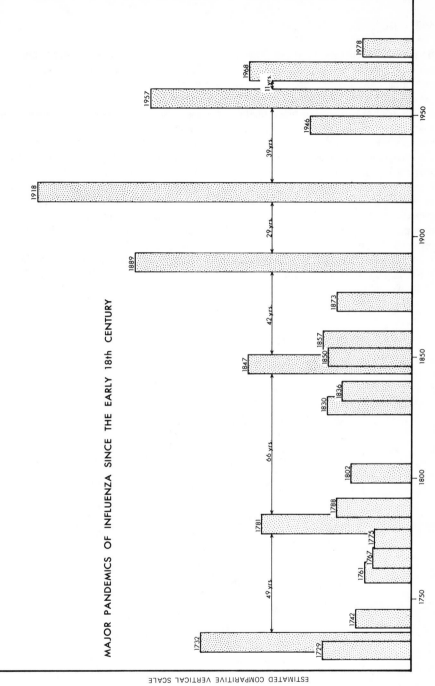

MAJOR PANDEMICS OF INFLUENZA SINCE THE EARLY 18th CENTURY

ESTIMATED COMPARATIVE VERTICAL SCALE

Fig. 70. Major pandemics and epidemics of Influenza in the world since the early 18th century (after Beveridge).

147

frequently occurring C type. The type A virus is particularly responsible for periodic worldwide pandemics. Due to antigenic variations in the A type virus, influenza can diffuse through human populations and attack persons who have developed antibodies through past viral infections.

These alterations take place in the surface protein of the virus (see Figure 71). Two kinds of surface spikes with separate functions exist on the surface of the virus. They are subject to change.[41] The more numerous, or hemagglutinin, are the mechanisms whereby the virus actually enters living cells to become absorbed. The second or enzymatic kinds of surface spikes are known as neuraminidase. These spikes attack the mucoprotein and are released in spittum or saliva, causing the spread of infection. In virological terms these spikes are referred to as H and N. As explained by Sir Charles Stuart-Harris, antigenic shift occurs in both H and N spikes.[42] This "drift" is a process whereby annual progressive change can take place. Every two to three years one epidemic succeeds another because of the change in the ratio between H and N. Major shifts can lead to worldwide pandemics (see Figure 72). From 1946 to 1957 it is

INFLUENZA VIRUS

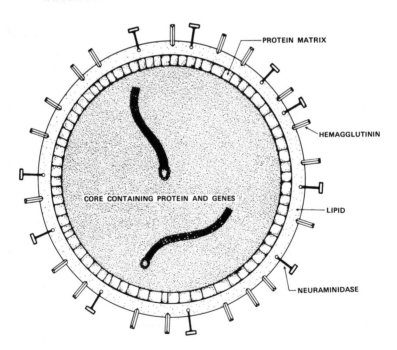

Fig. 71. An idealized diagram of an Influenza virus.

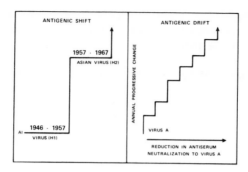

Fig. 72. An adaptation of the explanation of Stuart-Harris explaining antigenic shift and drift in Influenza viruses.

now known that the A virus giving rise to the diffusion of the disease was H1N1. By backtracking virologists have labeled influenza from 1920 to 1947 as H0N1. Following this pattern of antigenic shift, from 1957 to 1968 the prevailing A virus was H2N2. In 1968 shifts taking place gave rise to the H3N2 variant now prevalent in many parts of the world. More popular names for influenza, for example, "Asian," "Hong Kong," "Russian," "Spanish," and "swine flu," are usually the result of the *fons et origo* method in medicine of utilizing working names for diseases based on points of origin, or, in the case of influenza, places where it is estimated that epidemics began. At times such knowledge is not always exact, and locations early to report major outbreaks are used in this labeling process.

Now designated as $H_{sw}N1$ by Kilbourne, the great influenza epidemic of 1918 was responsible for from 10 to 20 million deaths, many of the victims healthy adults between 20 and 40 years of age.[43] Crosby's account of swine flu (or, Spanish influenza) indicates there was a first or primary wave of the disease which may have originated in the United States. He offers accounts of U.S. troops possibly spreading the disease to the World War I battlefront in Europe. Regardless of whether the disease originated in the United States, Spain, or as some have indicated, Sierra Leone, it quickly swept the world in two subsequent waves from the fall of 1918 to the spring of 1919. The disease was particularly severe because pneumonic complications often contributed to death.

Utilizing data obtained from Crosby's accountings of weekly cases of influenza reported within 50 major cities in the United States, it is possible to reconstruct a pattern of diffusion.[44] Weekly totals were transformed into percentiles, and a temporal distribution was determined for each location. This resulted in 50 logistic curves. Overall spatial patterns were then developed as response surfaces intended to approximate when different parts of the country reached the 25th,

50th, and 75th percentiles of the distributions. These surfaces shown within Figure 73 indicate the dramatic spread of influenza through the United States from east to west. These patterns verify Crosby's detailed textual accountings. Also, if this diffusion was indeed a second wave, there could have been some endemicity in Arkansas, Mississippi, and Lousiiana where there was very early and deep penetration.

The disease also penetrated the Upper Midwest with considerable speed. Some lag appears to have occurred in Ohio and Indiana, however. By the tenth week of

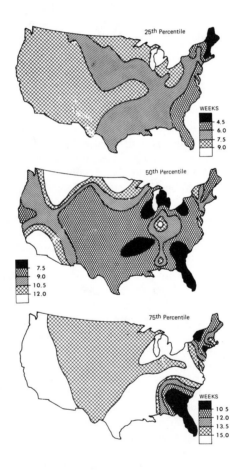

Fig. 73. The diffusion of Influenza in the United States in 1918.

the epidemic it had diffused well into the heartland of the United States. The 50th percentile surface indicates further penetration of the Pacific Coast. By the 20th week, influenza had spread into most of the country. Florida and Georgia continued to indicate relatively earlier reporting during the second two reconstructed phases. It is worthy of note that central portions of the country suffered prolonged effects of the epidemic. This particular method of mapping and measuring the disease diffusion proved to be useful when examining the very virulent $H_{sw}N1$ influenza.

The 1918 epidemic led to subsequent breakthroughs in the late 20s and early 1930s when the virus was identified.[45] For some reason that still mystifies many researchers, there was about a 40 year lag between the 1918 epidemic and the arrival of "Asian" influenza in 1957. Still, reference back to Figure 70 indicates that while the above time period may be considered interpandemic, the 1946 H1N1 strain was of epidemic proportion.

Much more is known about the origin and dispersal of the Asian influenza epidemic of 1957. Figure 74 shows that the virus probably originated in China in February 1957. By May of the same year it had spread to Japan, the Philippines, Indonesia, Australia, and India. The epidemic had diffused by August of 1957 to many other parts of the world. (The reader is reminded of Hunter and Young's analysis of the disease using mortality.) It is through the analysis of excessive mortality information that the true pandemic nature of influenza in 1957 can be understood. Experiences since 1918 had allowed epidemiologists to develop an average expected oscillation for normal cycles of influenza. Any observations in excess of this mortality can definitely be considered associated with epidemic influenza (see Eichhoff, Sherman, and Serfling).[46] Normally influenza is considered as a high morbidity–low mortality disease. When excessive deaths occur, for example, approximately 86,000 in 1957 in the United States alone, then the evidence is clear.

One strong indication of a pending influenza epidemic is not only excessive mortality but also time of occurrence. It is quite common for an epidemic to begin during the summer and spread very early in the fall. Figure 75, adapted from Osborn's work, shows how rapidly Asian flu spread through the United States in 1957.[47] This generalized pattern of diffusion indicates one path of spread from west to east and another northward along the Mississippi River complex. In July of 1957, Louisiana and California were reporting early cases. By August it had spread to adjacent areas including Florida. New areas of penetration also included New Mexico, Montana, and New York. The disease subsequently diffused into the country to ultimately encompass the Great Plains and Middle Atlantic by October of 1957.

Many epidemiologists have speculated that we are now in an interpandemic era, while others suggest that an epidemic is quite probable any time. With the appearance of the presumably new viral strain of A/New Jersey influenza (swine flu?) in 1976, the United States government launched a major innoculation program geared toward preventing an epidemic during the 1976–77 season. As with many mass innoculation programs, there were differences of opinion about the need for such measures.[48] Many simply thought that influenza was so well

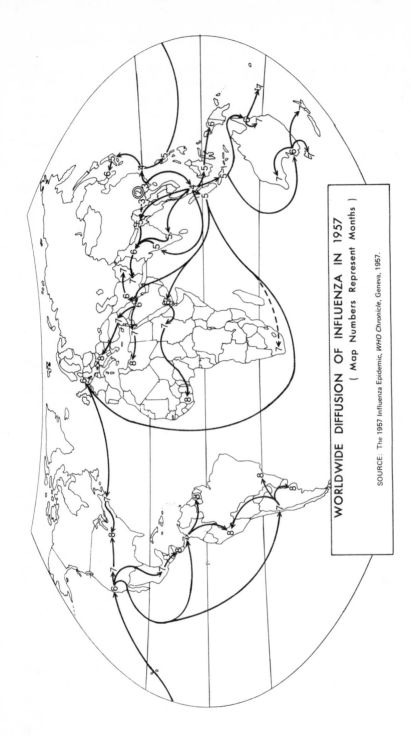

Fig. 74. The worldwide diffusion of "Asian" Influenza in 1957. The early penetration appeared to be on the West Coast and in the Gulf area.

152

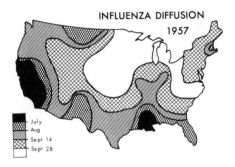

Fig. 75. A Generalized Depiction of Influenza Diffusion in the United States in 1957. The early penetration appeared to be on the West Coast and in the Gulf area.

"seeded" in the United States that a program would be of limited utility. In an attempt to control for H3N2 (Hong Kong) along with the new strain of influenza, the Center for Disease Control, with Congressional support, implemented a program involving both monovalent and bivalent innoculations. In the fall of 1976 the elderly were first to be innoculated. Younger adults were next. Some troublesome problems had developed. The program was halted because of some indications of possible complications in the form of varying degrees of reaction associated with the vaccine.

It cannot be stated, however, that the innoculation program was not successful. When actual influenza–pneumonia deaths are compared to expected for a five season period (see Figure 76), there is evidence of an epidemic trend from 1973-74 to 1975-76.[49] This was sufficient cause to launch the innoculation program. During the 1976-77 season, when mass innoculations were given, mortality was within expected limits. However, during the 1977-78 season, mortality attributed to influenza had unfortunately again exceeded the expected average. In light of the above development, it is extremely useful to examine in some detail the temporal and spatial distributions of influenza reporting within the United States during the most recent three seasons in an attempt to gain more knowledge about the medical geography of influenza in years of high and low mortality.

In a fashion similar to that utilized in detailing the 1918 epidemic, reporting for 120 cities (influenza-pneumonia mortality) was examined on the basis of weeks during which various locations reached different percentiles. Since these periods were not epidemic, the resultant spatial patterns are different from earlier findings. Preliminary analysis indicated that many parts of the country were "preseeded." It was necessary to view the 15th percentile of each distribution

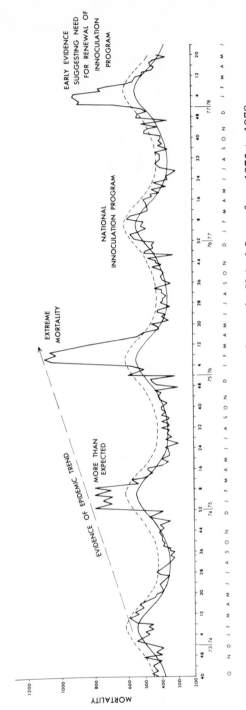

Fig. 76. Cycles of Influenza–Pneumonia mortality in the United States from 1973 to 1978.

along with those used previously. Sequences of maps (Figures 77, 78, and 79) containing the 15th, 25th, 50th, and 75th percentiles for the 120 cities during the three influenza seasons were constructed. Initially, wave-like national patterns were anticipated; however, this frequently did not result. Instead, regional shifts could be identified, and some extremely useful observations can be made pertaining to temporal distributions *within* different parts of the country. This is more apparent from one season to the next than within seasons. In other words, there appears to be a definite relationship between late penetration (75th percentile) during the end of one influenza season followed by very early reporting (15th percentile) the next season in adjacent locations.

As already indicated, excessive mortality during the 1975-76 influenza season was one reason for the innoculation program of 1976. Figure 77 shows the changing mortality patterns during that season. The 15th percentile map, or early reporting, is an indication of when particular parts of the country reached this cumulative proportion from the 5th to 11th weeks (the fall of 1975). Those places attaining the 15th percentile very early included parts of the Midwest and southern Atlantic coast. The Great Plains area showed fairly early reporting, along with south-central California. Those parts of the country reaching the 15th percentile later, or during the 10th and 11th weeks, included large portions of Texas, the Southwest, the Pacific Northwest, northern New England, and parts of the Mid-Atlantic area. The 25th percentile pattern gives some indication of diffusion within broad regions of the country, but forms of lag also show up. For example, the Midwestern part of the country seems to have been an endemic core area. The same can be stated for the New York area and parts of California. Conversely, parts of the Pacific Northwest and the mountain areas of the country along with Texas and the Carolina coast continued to show a later arrival at the 25th percentile (approximately during the 14th and 15th weeks). A pattern of regular diffusion from points of origin does not show up throughout the entire United States, and this should not be expected during a nonepidemic year in spite of the excessive mortality.

By the time the 50th percentile was reached in many parts of the country, a trend emerged wherein more and more parts of the Eastern United States reached that measure sooner than parts of the Western United States. By the spring of 1976, influenza was on the wane. The map showing the 75th percentile gives some indication of earlier arrivals at that phase in the East and later arrivals in the West. Particular attention should be paid to those parts of the country attaining the 75th percentile late in the spring of 1976. Included were parts of the Middle Atlantic, eastern Ohio, the Gulf Coast, the Great Plains, the Southwest, and the Northwest. The pattern containing 75th percentile data would not be nearly so meaningful without a comparison of the patterns developed from measuring the 15th percentile during the fall of 1976, the beginning of the next season (Figure 78).

In spite of the national innoculation program, parts of the country with late attainment of the 75th percentile in the spring of 1976 were some of the first parts of the country to show early reporting the following autumn. Parts of the country reaching the 15th percentile between the 4th and 9th weeks of the

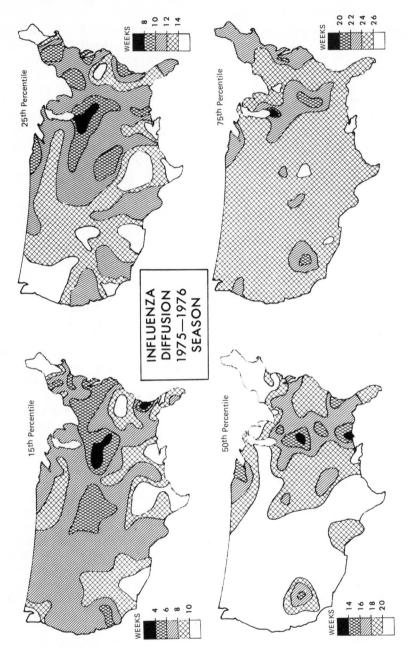

Fig. 77. Influenza diffusion in the United States during the 1975–1976 Season.

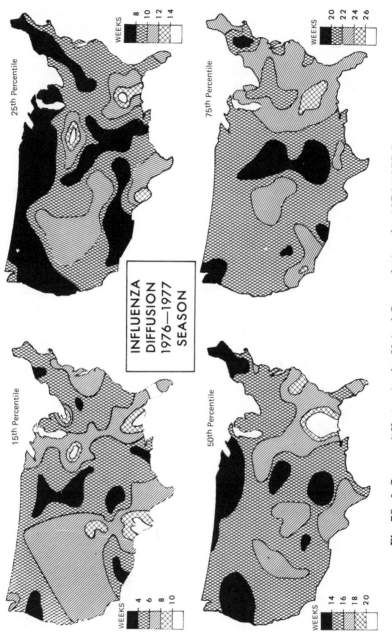

15th Percentile

25th Percentile

50th Percentile

75th Percentile

INFLUENZA
DIFFUSION
1976—1977
SEASON

WEEKS
4
6
8
10

WEEKS
8
10
12
14

WEEKS
14
16
18
20

WEEKS
20
22
24
26

Fig. 78. Influenza diffusion in the United States during the 1976–1977 Season.

157

season included the Pacific Northwest, parts of the Southwest, the western Gulf Coast area, parts of Ohio, and upper New York state. This pattern immediately gives rise to the possibility that the virus had summered over in these areas in such a manner as to cause early outbreaks in the fall of 1976. In other words, it can be hypothesized that not all susceptible victims acquired influenza during the waning phase, and as soon as the temperatures dropped in the fall the areas already mentioned were some of the first parts of the country to demonstrate early reporting. Subsequent spatial "pulsations" of influenza during the 1976-77 season are shown within Figure 78 in the form of 25th, 50th, and 75th percentile maps. In general, these patterns show regional progressions of reporting during the 25th and 50th percentiles in areas adjacent to the earliest reporting. By the spring of 1977 regions of the country showing lags in reaching the 75th percentile consisted of parts of the Atlantic Coast, the extreme Southwestern part of the United States and a large area in the Southeast.

Once again the pattern of inverse associations, i.e., lags in reporting during one spring followed by early reporting during the next, showed up when the reporting for the 1977-78 season was examined (see Figure 79). For example, locations with more reporting during the 15th percentile (from the 5th through 9th weeks of the fall of 1977) are many of those places that showed lags during the spring of 1977. They included parts of the Southeast, southern California, and large parts of the Western Plains. It is also of importance that many regions reaching the 75th percentile early in the spring of 1977 showed later attainment of the 15th and subsequent percentiles during the 1977-78 season. These regularities appear to be systematic in spite of reported mortality figures from one season to the next (see Figure 76).

While no clearly defined wave-like penetrations of the country were indicated in the analysis of the three influenza seasons, it is worthy of note that much can be learned about oscillations and spatial pulsations of influenza within a country during nonepidemic years. In spite of the lowered mortality during the 1976-77 season, the general pattern of early reporting one season followed by late reporting the next indicates that certain kinds of spatial-temporal microscale diffusion is operating within regions of the country during high and low incidence years. While this finding is extremely useful and should be monitored over time in perhaps even greater detail, it cannot be assumed that yet another new strain of influenza will not develop and diffuse throughout the country in some rapid and regular fashion. This could happen by linear diffusion, radial diffusion, and hierarchical diffusion simultaneously.

At the time of this writing the influenza problem is far from solved. According to Webster and Laver there are several ways in which viruses can change.[50] These include mutation, adaptation, and hybridization. It is not only possible for new strains to develop, but there is also the chance of recycling of antigens which could lead to future pandemics. Influenza A is known to be established in lower animals and birds. According to Kilbourne, one form of the movement of viruses appears to be from man to mammals and birds.[51] It is hypothetically possible that as one viral strain victimizing man declines, and starts to show up in animals, forms of mutation, adaptation, and hybridization

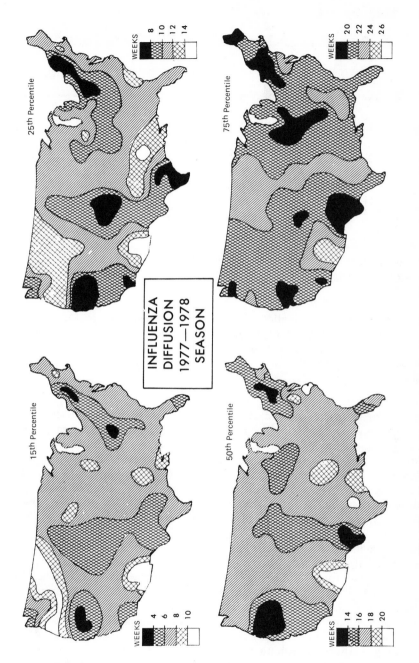

Fig. 79. Influenza diffusion in the Untied States during the 1977-1978 Season.

159

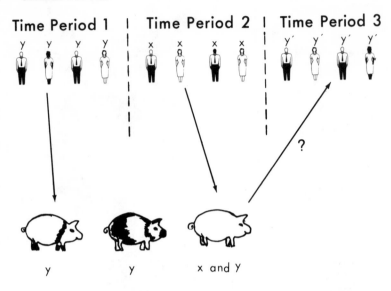

Fig. 80. An adaptation of Kilbourne's explanation of the possibility of two kinds of Influenza virus moving from humans to animals to combine and possibly return to humans during three periods of time.

may take place in animals and eventually a new virus can move back to man. Figure 80 helps in illustrating this possibility as explained by Kilbourne. In what Kilbourne calls a rare event, it is possible for a human influenza virus (indicated as strain Y) to infect a domestic animal and subsequently become established within those animals. Another strain, X (similar to the development of the Hong Kong strain) begins to occur in man. If this strain is also passed to animals, it is possible that another kind of virus combining traits of the two can develop. Another rare event might consist of the transmittal of this kind of virus (X and Y) back to man in the form of Y'. Assuming Y' is "swine flu," or perhaps any virulent strain, it could indeed give rise to a worldwide pandemic. Some researchers have speculated that so long as one kind of virus is strong, it is difficult for new forms to develop.[52] Given the disappearance of a certain kind of virus, many susceptible victims could be seriously affected by the diffusion of a "new" kind of influenza. From a geographical point of view it is clearly important that various strains of virus be analyzed temporally and spatially on a regular basis. Important kinds of information pertaining to locations of outbreaks can lead to early implementation of control measures and hopefully result in preventing an epidemic similar to that of 1918. This is one application of medical geography that has the potential of saving countless lives.

NOTES

[1] A. Hirsch. *Handbook of Geographical and Historical Pathology.* 3 vols. (Trans., C. Creighten, Jr.) London: New Sydenham Society (1883–1886).

[2] See Chapter 1, note 15.

[3] J. M. Hunter. "River Blindness in Nangodi, Northern Ghana: A Hypothesis of Cyclical Advance and Retreat," *The Geographical Review,* Vol. 56 (1966), pp. 398–416.

[4] See Chapter 3, note 11.

[5] See Chapter 3, note 8.

[6] S. N. De. *Cholera, Its Pathology and Pathogenesis.* Edinburgh: Oliver and Boyd (1961), pp. 1–72.

[7] See Chapter 1, note 15.

[8] G. F. Pyle. "The Diffusion of Cholera in the United States in the Nineteenth Century," *Geographical Analysis,* Vol. 1 (1969), pp. 59–75.

[9] Richard Gallagher. *Diseases That Plague Modern Man: A History of Ten Communicable Diseases.* Dobbs Ferry, N.Y.: Oceana Publications (1969).

[10] Center for Disease Control. "Hepatitis Surveillance," Report 40, March 1977, Atlanta, Georgia.

[11] P. F. Wehrle, J. Posch, K. H. Richter, and D. A. Henderson. "An Airborne Outbreak of Smallpox in a German Hospital and Its Significance with Respect to Other Recent Outbreaks in Europe," *Bulletin, World Health Organization,* Vol. 43 (1970), pp. 669–679.

[12] Melville R. Klauber and Juan J. Angulo. "Three Tests for Randomness of Attack of Social Groups During an Epidemic," *American Journal of Epidemiology,* Vol. 104 (1976), pp. 212–218.

[13] Juan J. Angulo, Peter Haggett, and Carlos A. A. Pederneiras. "Variola Minor in Braganca Paulista County, 1956: A Trend-Surface Analysis," *American Journal of Epidemiology,* Vol. 105 (1977), pp. 272–280.

[14] K. L. Gould, K. L. Herrman, and J. J. Witte. "The Epidemiology of Measles in the U.S. Trust Territory of the Pacific Islands," *American Journal of Public Health,* Vol. 61 (1971), pp. 1602–1613.

[15] E. G. Knox. "Epidemics of Rare Diseases," *British Medical Bulletin,* Vol. 27 (1971), pp. 43–47.

[16] These concepts are summarized by Ronald Abler, John S. Adams, and Peter Gould. *Spatial Organization: The Geographer's View of the World.* Englewood Cliffs: Prentice-Hall (1971), Chapter 11. Also see Torsten Hagerstrand. "Aspects of the Spatial Structure of Social Communication," Regional Science Association, Paper 14, Cracow Congress, 1965.

[17] Jui-Cheng Huang and Peter Gould. "Diffusion in an Urban Hierarchy: The Case of Rotary Clubs," *Economic Geography,* Vol. 50 (1974), pp. 333–340.

[18] Richard Morrill. "The Negro Ghetto: Problems and Alternatives," *Geographical Review,* Vol. 55 (1965), pp. 339–361.

[19] Ronald Abler, John S. Adams, and Peter Gould, op. cit., also Torsten Hagerstrand, op. cit.

[20] Lawrence A. Brown and E. G. Moore. "Diffusion Research: A Perspective," in C. Board, R. J. Chorley, Peter Haggett, and D. R. Stoddart (eds.), *Progress in Geography* (Ch. 4). London: Edward Arnold (1969), pp. 120–157.

[21] Torsten Hagerstrand. *The Propagation of Innovation Waves: Lund Studies in Geography,* Series B, No. 4. Lund: Gleerup (1952).

[22] Stafford Beer. *Management Science: The Business Use of Operations Research.* Garden City: Doubleday (1968).

[23] Judith Meyer. "A Typology of Diffusion and Adoption Processes," *Proceedings, Association of American Geographers*, Vol. 7 (1975), pp. 146–150.

[24] Brian J. L. Berry. "Cities as Systems Within Systems of Cities," *Papers of the Regional Science Association*, Vol. 13 (1964), pp. 147–164.

[25] Paul Ove Pedersen. "Innovation Diffusion Within and Between Urban Systems," *Geographical Analysis*, Vol. 2 (1970), pp. 203–254.

[26] Brian J. L. Berry. "The Geography of the United States in the Year 2000," *Transactions of the Institute of the British Geographers*, Vol. 51 (1970), pp. 21–53. See also Brian J. L. Berry, Edgar C. Conkling, and D. Michael Ray. *The Geography of Economic Systems*. Englewood Cliffs: Prentice-Hall (1976), pp. 492–494.

[27] *Economic Geography*, Vol. 50, No. 4 (1974) and Vol. 51, No. 3 (1975).

[28] Peter Haggett. *Locational Analysis in Human Geography*. New York: St. Martins (1966), pp. 56–60.

[29] Peter Haggett. "Hybridizing Alternative Models of an Epidemic Diffusion Process," *Economic Geography*, Vol. 52 (1976), pp. 136–146.

[30] John W. Florin. *Death in New England: Regional Variations in Mortality*. Chapel Hill: University of North Carolina, Department of Geography (1971).

[31] Kwame Mayer Kwofie. "A Spatio-Temporal Analysis of Cholera Diffusion in Western Africa," *Economic Geography*, Vol. 52 (1976), pp. 127–135.

[32] Robert Stock. *Cholera in Africa*. London: International African Institute (1976).

[33] A. A. Brownlea. "An Urban Ecology of Infectious Disease: City of Greater Wollongong–Shell Harbour," *Australian Geographer*, Vol. 10 (1967), pp. 169–187.

[34] Neil D. McGlashan. "Viral Hepatitis in Tasmania," *Scoial Science and Medicine (Medical Geography)*, Vol. 11 (1977), pp. 731–744.

[35] John M. Hunter and Johnathan C. Young. "Diffusion of Influenza in England and Wales," *Annals* of the Association of American Geographers, Vol. 61 (1971), pp. 637–653.

[36] Richard Gallagher, op. cit., pp. 39–54.

[37] E. D. Kilbourne. "The Influenza Viruses and Influenza–An Introduction" in Edwin D. Kilbourne (ed.), *The Influenza Viruses and Influenza*. New York: Academic Press (1957), pp. 1–14.

[38] Ibid.

[39] W. I. B. Beveridge. *Influenza: The Last Great Plague: An Unfinished Story of Discovery*. New York: Prodist (1977).

[40] R. E. Shope. *Journal of Experimental Medicine*, Vol. 54 (1931), pp. 373–375.

[41] Purnell W. Choppin and Richard W. Compans. "The Structure of Influenza Virus" in Edwin D. Kilbourne (ed.), *The Influenza Viruses and Influenza*. New York: Academic Press (1975), pp. 15–51.

[42] Charles Stuart-Harris. "The Influenza Problem," *Medical Laboratory Technology*, Vol. 32 (1975), pp. 161–169; and *Influenza and Other Virus Infections of the Respiratory Tract*. Baltimore: Williams and Williams (1961).

[43] Alfred W. Crosby, Jr. *Epidemic and Peace, 1918*. Westport, Conn.: Greenwood Press (1976). See also June E. Osborn (ed.), *History, Science, and Politics: Influenza in America 1918-1976*. New York: Prodist (1977).

[44] Alfred W. Grosby, Jr., op. cit., pp. 60–61, 65.

[45] A. J. Rhodes and C. E. VanRooyen. *Textbook of Virology*. 5th ed. Baltimore: Williams and Wilkins (1968).

[46] Theodore C. Eickhoff, Ida L. Sherman, and Robert E. Serfling. "Observations on Excess Mortality Associated with Epidemic Influenza," *Journal American Medical Association*, Vol. 176 (1961), pp. 776–782.

[47] June E. Osborn, op. cit.

[48] J. Donald Millar and June E. Osborn. "Precursors of the Scientific Decision-Making Process Leading to the 1976 National Immunization Campaign" in June E. Osborn (ed.), *History, Science, and Politics: Influenza in America 1918-1976.* New York: Prodist (1977), pp. 15-27.

[49] Center for Disease Control, Atlanta, Georgia. *Influenza Surveillance Reports,* 1974-1977.

[50] Robert G. Webster and W. Graeme Lauer. "Antigenic Variation of Influenza Viruses" in Edwin D. Kilbourne (ed.), *The Influenza Viruses and Influenza.* New York: Academic Press (1975), pp. 270-310.

[51] E. D. Kilbourne. "Epidemiology of Influenza" in Edwin D. Kilbourne (ed.), *The Influenza Viruses and Influenza.* New York: Academic Press (1975), pp. 483-538.

[52] Louis Weinstein. "Influenza—1918, A Revisit?" *The New England Journal of Medicine,* Vol. 294 (1976), pp. 1058-1062.

Chapter 6

VARIABLE METHODS
OF ASSOCIATION

Writing in 1967 on geographical evidence in medical hypotheses, McGlashan stated that geographers can offer much in the way of contributing to medical knowledge through what he generally termed "associative occurrences."[1] He contended that it is necessary to make a distinction between physical environmental elements and socioeconomic or cultural environments. McGlashan also called on geographers to develop quantitative analyses associating variable elements possibly contributing to spatial variations of disease occurrence. Until the late 1960s and early 1970s, one of the criticisms that could be leveled against geographers dealing in such matters pertained to the use of extremely gross generalizations made on the basis of comparisons of different cartographic patterns, as indicated in Chapter 3.

A multiplicity of issues must be addressed in undertaking this kind of endeavor. There are questions of different scientific methods in the social and natural sciences. For example, the geographer might have the tendency to attempt exhaustive mapping of different diseases, followed with a quantitative analysis of different variables reported for similar units of observation. Conversely, partially due to training and intent of such studies, the epidemiologist is more prone to extract different kinds of samples from larger populations and draw conclusions. Additional issues influencing methods of analysis consist of type of disease, geographic scale, methods of designing hypotheses, and preferences for particular nonparametric and parametric methods of analyses.

In medical geography, associative analyses must take a more holistic rather than dichotomous approach when undertaking such endeavors. While it is useful to attempt to identify either physical or social environments, it is not always practical to make such distinctions. Environment as a term should be broadly defined in studies of medical geography, and the entire concept of environment can be viewed as a cultural continuum ranging from the most simple to more complex cultures.[2] It is true that generalized distinctions are made even when viewing environment from this broader perspective. One example is (Figure 4 in Chapter 2) Dever's general interpretation of cycles of disease patterns characteristic of agrarian cultural influences compared with disease patterns of a more chronic nature characteristic of industrial and post-industrial societies.[3] It should be understood that there is an entire range of cycles from one of these extremes to the other. Still, it is useful to compare the different fertility ratios and the types of chronic diseases more characteristic of advanced societies and problems of malnutrition, infectious diseases and parasitic ailments in less economically developed cultures. Clearly, in many countries both of these extreme conditions exist, perhaps in the form of urban and rural differences in some cases. Combinations of patterns between the two extremes should be expected.

Availability of information also varies with different cultures. Much health-related information useful for spatial analysis, particularly in the United States, is in the form of mortality reporting rather than morbidity. The investigator working in medicogeographic studies in less advanced locations is often required to accomplish extensive field work to extract samples for comparative purposes because the data are not available in any other fashion. In the latter case, it is often necessary and advisable to utilize nonparametric statistical methods of analysis due to constraints built into sampling techniques. Variable kinds of mortality and (sometimes) morbidity information obtained in more advanced and industrialized societies often appears to be more amenable to parametric methods of statistical analysis. Regardless of the geographic area under investigation, the health researcher is often limited to use of available information.

Existing associative occurrence studies range from some of a speculative nature to others attempting forms of statistical explanation. The latter are often in the form of comparative testing of illness rates by age, sex, and social class in some form of causal association. One underlying issue with many of these analyses, as with any research design, consists of selection of methods of analysis. Methodological frameworks range from simple chi-square testing for significance to the use of complex multivariate explanations. To some extent research from different disciplines tends to become "formulized" in the sense that certain kinds of statistical methods are preferred over others. Problems may arise when health data that can be tested parametrically are only examined with nonparametric tests of significance. As explained later in this chapter, the same kinds of information may show little or no significance when utilizing chi-square tests, but when they are tested with parametric methods, there is significance. The opposite is also true.

Some Areas of Interpretive Difficulty

In a recent review of the use of data analysis techniques in biomedical research, Vargo found that while there is increased use of quantification in associative comparisons, research methodologies are often not well designed. There is a greater tendency for misinterpretation of statistical results as well as for actual commission of errors in some examples.[4] Probable errors include sampling problems, control errors, improper formulations, miscalculations, and spurious conclusions. The validity of any such associative studies basically depends on the reasonable and correct use of "best-fitting" techniques.

As indicated within Chapter Three, the researcher embarking upon studies in medical geography must constantly be cognizant of geographic scale. Particular conclusions that might be reached at the international scale may not be substantiated at a microgeographic scale, and the reverse, of course, is also possible. Between these scales there may also be a continuum of statistical explanation. At the international and often national scales, one recurring general underlying theme is that variable levels of economic development which correspond to general cultural patterns correlate with disease measures. The factor analyses used in Chapter Three are intended to show disease clusters, but the same general association is *implied*. In their explanation of worldwide health problems, Joseph, Koch-Weser, and Wallace offer an easily understandable approach to this continuum of associations.[5]

Burbank's work on cancer distributions in the United States contains some implication of disease occurrence differentials due to variable regional economies, but it is not possible to make generalized urban-rural distinctions because of the state data base.[6] More recently the *National Cancer Atlas of the United States* has offered further background information by depicting differences at the county level.[7] Still, without a nationwide tumor registry, detailed county morbidity analysis is somewhat difficult. With the information contained in the *National Cancer Atlas,* research utilizing statistical testing methods to explain unexpected regional concentrations of different kinds of cancers is quite possible.

Much remains to be done also in terms of mathematically testing cultural explanations. For example, in a geographical analysis of lung cancer in the Soviet Union, where a turmor registry exists, Bogovski, Purde, and Rahu considered generalized ethnocultural explanations when viewing the epidemiology of lung cancer, but other factors were deemed more important.[8] They found that in the Soviet Far East, standardized mortality for lung cancer from 1959 to 1969 was higher in rural than in urban areas. The same was true in the Karelian S.S.R., however. They attributed this circumstance to climatic instead of cultural differences. In the Rostow area there was a very high rate of cancer morbidity in coal mining areas, as would be expected. While it might be possible to formally test for cultural determinants in a country with such ethnic diversity as the Soviet Union, it is extremely difficult due to intervening climatic and economic variables.

AN EPIDEMIOLOGICAL BASIS FOR ASSOCIATIVE STUDIES

Epidemiological knowledge is absolutely essential to studies in medical geography. Without the necessary background about epidemiological elements contributing to the occurrence of any particular disease, the medical geographer may be confronted with many maps and statistics and little or no meaningful explanation. Epidemiological information pertaining to geographic factors and disease is found in the form of simple to very complex works. For purposes of spatial analysis, an inherent weakness in many epidemiological studies is that cartographic exercises accompanying explanations are often far too elementary. (As already indicated in Chapter 3, the Poisson distribution approach espoused by McGlashan can do much to enhance many epidemiological studies.) Conversely, the rich literature of epidemiology can be used much more by researchers in the area of medical geography than it was in the past.

From Environment to Culture

For example, with reference to environmentally-oriented disease ecological approaches, Kafuko and Burkitt contended in a 1970 publication that the distribution of Burkitt's lymphoma may be "related" to malaria endemicity.[9] Much of the evidence used to support that hypothesis was based on laboratory tests and a clinical sample. However, their geographical evidence consisted of a "lymphoma belt" defined earlier by Burkitt in Africa based on generalized climate and altitude (see Figure 36 in Chapter 3). In the 1970 study their hypothesis was that a biological agent, possibly an insect vector, may also be responsible for the lymphoma. With an awareness of inconsistencies in explaining the occurrence of lymphoma, Kafuko and Burkitt used East Africa as a geographical area for their associative analysis. Samples of lymphoma patients were examined on the basis of age and disease severity, and subsequent comparisons were made with the geographical occurrence of malaria. While they found a higher incidence of both Burkitt's lymphoma and malarial infection, a close association between the two maladies could only be presumed.

A similar approach was taken by Campbell in a geographic macroscale discussion of the epidemiology of multiple sclerosis.[10] The contribution of Campbell is of particular interest to the medical geographer because it offers an agenda for future research. Campbell explains how multiple sclerosis appears to be remarkably uncommon in occurrence within Africa as well as Japan. He futher states that no definite explanation of variations in multiple sclerosis is offered by simple contentions of latitudinal banding; thus suggesting that climate is not an important explanatory factor. Campbell contends instead that the occurrence of multiple sclerosis appears to be highly localized in different parts of the world. One possible explanation may be trace elements in soils, particularly lead and copper. As with the example·of goitre mentioned earlier in this book, there does appear to be some association with settlement patterns in glaciated areas. In reviewing some of the literature Campbell points out how the occurrence of multiple sclerosis may be explained by dietary intake. There appear to be parts of the world, Iceland and South Africa, for example, wherein the incidence of the disease may be associated with ingestion of fatty tissue, particularly from sheep. It is of interest that according to Campbell, multiple sclerosis cuts across various socioeconomic levels. Campbell also indicates that the incidence of multiple sclerosis appears to be higher in certain rural parts of the world than in more urbanized areas. While some have suggested possible viral linkages to the disease, Campbell nonetheless leans toward dietary explanations. The most important statement made by Campbell is, "It would appear that some important link in the chain of facts about multiple sclerosis is missing." This admission is what presents the challenge for future research in medical geography.

For some of the reasons mentioned above, there is little question that it is easier to develop studies of associative occurrence utilizing mortality data obtained within more technologically advanced nations. The epidemiological literature virtually abounds with such studies. Many, but not all of these studies, are accomplished in a very traditional epidemiological mode: (1) mortality data are obtained from specific populations; (2) various crude, age-specific, age-adjusted, and standardized mortality ratios are determined for population samples; and (3) descriptive trends are developed for further analysis. Quite often the epidemiological researcher's hypothesis is that the incidence of a particular kind of mortality is on the increase; this hypothesis is followed by tables and graphs and occasional significance tests offered as proof. In other instances the decreasing occurrence over time of particular ailments is depicted in a similar fashion. The information is valuable but explanations are often merely speculative.

In 1972, Creagan and Fraumeni of the Epidemiology Branch of the National Cancer Institute (United States) published a comparative analysis of cancer mortality among American Indians from 1950-1967.[11] The study was of particular interest because, with the exception of gall bladder cancer, the development of carcinomas among American Indians, both male and female, has been lower than the national rate. Utilizing data files of the National Center for Health Statistics, they compared cause of death by sex, race, age, county, and state. Comparisons were drawn among white and nonwhite males, white and nonwhite females and American Indian males and females. The comparisons were accomplished utilizing standardized mortality ratios (observed deaths compared to expected). The results of the study indicate how American Indians generally manifest lower cancer rates for most histological sites. Creagan and Fraumeni attributed this phenomenon to higher than national diabetes rates among American Indians. The geographic implications of this finding are many. Could this relationship be due to culture? Diet? Blood groups? The topic requires detailed geographical research.

As explained within Chapter 7 of this book, several medical geographers have developed useful methodologies for associative analysis within hospital-based data. Such opportunities exist because of the availability of this kind of epidemiological information. Johansson's compilation of statistics about myocardial infarction in Malmo from 1960 to 1968 is an example of the kind of information useful for beginning analyses of particular chronic and degenerative diseases.[12] In this instance, more than 3,000 patients suffering from a "heart attack" were analyzed. Johansson stated that the study population was of particular importance because most of the inhabitants of Malmo are served by a single, major hospital. When this is the case, more uniform epidemiological data are available. After subgrouping patients by age and sex, Johansson was able to make some useful comparisons. For example, the case fatality rate for the time period under study was approximately one-third of the sample. Obesity was present in about 14% of the patients. More than 7% of the male patients and almost 13% of the female patients had an earlier diagnosis of diabetes. Hypertension was diagnosed in about 7% of the males and 15% of the females. Only 6% of the female and 7% of the male patients had a past history of heart disease. Seventy-seven percent of the patients under study had not previously had a myocardial infarct, while 18% had at least one. While Johansson did not offer any formal hypotheses or statistical tests, he provided information which when compared to other locations is the sort required for comparative geographical analyses of heart disease in general.

A wide variety of epidemiological studies can be used as important background information for further analysis, as is evidenced in a study published in 1963 by Nyman Scotch, pertaining to sociocultural factors related to Zulu hypertension in South Africa.[13] Scotch used samples of 548 Zulus in an urban area and 505 in a rural area for comparative analysis. Utilizing chi-square testing with 4 X 4 contingency tables, Scotch found that many of the variables utilized in other studies pertaining to stress were not statistically significant in the Zulu samples. He did find out, however, that urban Zulu populations showed higher mean blood pressures than those from rural areas. Also through the use of chi-square testing, statistical significance between hypertension and age, sex, obesity, martial status, and church attendance were identified. Unlike many other epidemiological findings, Scotch claimed that hypertension is multifaceted and cannot be explained by any single variable in a general association. Of additional interest was Scotch's statement that the more rapidly the Zulu acculturated to urban society, the less likely they were to suffer from hypertension.

And a Return to Environment

In a 1970 study, Haber and Lipkovic analyzed the incidence of thyroid cancer in Oahu, Hawaii, in relation to environmental factors.[14] They selected Hawaii as a study location because of what they considered a "unique and heterogeneous racial mixture of peoples." Data were obtained from hospital medical records and pathology departments. Haber and Lipkovic utilized standard measurement methods in converting cases to crude age specific and age standardized incidence rates. According to results from their sampling techniques, the incidence of thyroid cancer in women in Hawaii is one of the highest in the world, and it is very high among men. They attemped to explain the high incidence of thyroid cancer in Oahu populations as somehow associated with the environment. It was explained that the two major environmental factors previously considered in helping to explain thyroid cancer were iodine and ionizing radiation. Since they could find no evidence of iodine deficiency in Hawaii, the general conclusion was made that the higher incidence of thyroid cancer must be related to ionizing radiation. This hypothesized association is worthy of scientific follow-up, especially since Haber and Lipkovic offered no statistical testing in support of their finding. Ionizing radiation probably does have a major role in contributing to thyroid cancer in Hawaii. The implications of this study are of geographic significance because one possible environmental hazard was selected as a contributing cause to a particular kind of cancer.

In a different kind of epidemiological study of cancer in relation to sources of drinking water in Ohio, Kuzma, Kuzma, and Buncher performed an analysis of covariance using age, sex, and race-adjusted cancer rates (1950 to 1969), population variables, measures of urbanization, income, and occupation.[15] In what is one of the first of such attempts, the authors obtained information from the Environmental Protection Agency (EPA) pertaining to sources of drinking water, i.e., surface water or ground water, for 88 counties in Ohio. Previous EPA studies had indicated that certain concentrations of carcinogenic chemicals are higher in surface water supplies than in those obtained from wells. On the basis of land area served, Ohio counties adjacent to Lake Erie and the Ohio River were among those identified as using surface water primarily. The authors found significantly higher stomach and bladder cancer rates in parts of Ohio served by mostly surface water sources. Also, overall cancer rates were significantly higher in counties relying on surface water supplies. Certain histologic sites did not prove to be significant. They included breast and lung cancer. One of the research problems encountered by Kuzma, Kuzma, and Buncher was extreme difficulty in controlling for urbanization and occupation groups. However, the use of covariance analysis in such investigations is essential for testing purposes.

In another study of cancer variations in relation to environmental influences, MacDonald analyzed mortality data for a 30-year period (1940–1969) by sex and ethnicity in 15 subareas of the city of Houston.[16] She defined data collection subareas of Houston on the basis of air pollution information. Since there are almost always more census tracts than air pollution data collection stations in cities, the researcher is forced to define subareas in such a fashion. Houston is a rapidly growing urban center heavily reliant on petrochemical industries, with seven oil refineries in the metropolitan area. Unlike many other environmentally-oriented air pollution studies, MacDonald effectively used maps in analyzing the annual distribution of air pollutants within Houston. Age-adjusted mortality rates were determined by white, nonwhite, and Spanish surnamed groups within the city for total cancer, heart disease, and stroke. Expected findings, such as overall higher rates among nonwhites and Spanish surnamed populations, were identified. In an actual comparison of cancer rates among all groups in relation to measured pollution, MacDonald found that in parts of the city with extreme pollution, cancer rates were indeed higher, even when considering adjustments by population subgroups. She raises an additional issue of interest to the medical geographer. In some instances pollution data appeared to be "anomalous;" for example, areas with relatively high pollution have only moderate cancer rates. Accounting for variable wind direction and velocity was attempted, but it was extremely difficult to apply many conventional statistical tests because of differences in geographic units of observation utilized in obtaining demographic and pollution data.

Epidemiological studies explain causation by applying a variety of approaches in terms of hypothesis testing, kinds of statistical techniques and data gathering procedures. Many geographic explanations are suggested, particularly of an environmental nature. One of the paradoxes in medical geography is that many of the associative techniques utilized in epidemiological research are not adopted often in studies of disease ecology. Conversely, many studies pertaining to the environment accomplished by epidemiologists and other health researchers tend to define the concept in an extremely general fashion. Recently, Melinda Meade has successfully coped with this paradox by explaining methods of disease-ecological research that call for epidemiological considerations.[17] Similar to many of those discussed above, Meade's analytical framework can be considered as a model to follow in helping close the gap between medical geography and epidemiology. Until this is successfully accomplished, parallel but separate research trends will continue.

THE PARALLEL GEOGRAPHIC PATH

The results of long-term studies by Sakamoto-Momiyama and her colleagues at the Meteorological Society of Japan parallel epidemiological findings, especially in the area of associative environmental research. A 1975 study by Momiyama et al. is an excellent methodological example.[18] In this analysis of infant mortality in relation to climatic variations they show how seasonal peaks in infant mortality have been changing over time within Japan. Earlier studies showed extremely high infant mortality in very cold winter months, with a minor peak in warm months. The 1975 investigation indicated that infant mortality rates have recently been lowered within Japan during cold months, but that mortality in warm months has increased over the past decade. The result is a bimodal infant mortality rate. As in past studies accomplished by Momiyama and her colleagues, statistical significance could be found between extreme hot and cold temperature peaks and infant mortality. Furthermore, geographic variations in infant mortality from one part of the country could be identified. Additionally, different patterns of variation showed up in 1964 when compared to 1971. The latter finding is extremely important to the researcher examining spatial patterns of variation from one region of a country to another over time, because there is no guarantee that similar patterns will hold true temporally.

In a comparison of childhood lead poisoning and seasonality, Hunter demonstrated how lead poisoning tends to peak during summers, particularly in more industrialized urban places.[19] Hunter also identified lead concentrations as generally localized in older parts of settled areas and along traffic routes. He further demonstrated that while climatic factors were seasonally influencing lead levels, solar radiation also plays an important role. In other words, pica and lead ingestion can be considered year-round behavioral traits; but severe manifestations of childhood lead poisoning show definite summer peaks. Given at least the propensity for lead poisoning to vary seasonally, Hunter offers an integrative model to be utilized by researchers in understanding this seasonality.

Caprio, Margulis, and Joselow further demonstrated geographic differences in lead absorption in children with an analysis of residential location in relation to the probability of air-lead pollution.[20] Utilizing nonparametric statistical testing, Caprio, Margulis, and Joselow found that there were significant differences in affected children in relation to residential distance from major highways. Utilizing data obtained from sampling in Newark, New Jersey, they discovered a much higher proportion of affected children living within 100 feet of major urban thoroughfares. A fairly regular distance-decay relationship could be identified with distance away from major thoroughfares and decreasing amounts of lead levels in children tested. Thus, proximity to traffic can be considered a major problem in what definitely appears to be a summer disease. In another study, this one in East Orange, New Jersey, Margulis examined pediatric lead poisoning in relation to age of housing.[21] As would be expected, higher rates of childhood lead poisoning were found in parts of East Orange with older housing.

Condition of housing, age of structures, urban deterioration and many other factors have been brought into play in analyses of urban health hazards. In a 1974 study of environmental change in Detroit from 1961–1971, Lewis and Chadzynski developed an appraisal of environmental change in relation to health hazard in Detroit.[22] They noted a gradual aging of neighborhoods from the central city moving outward in a westerly direction over time. Lewis and Chadzynski claimed on the basis of cartographic comparisons that one of the key indicators of health problems in Detroit is trash. The prevalence of rubble was mapped over time and trash also increased in a westward direction outward from the center of the city. In a similar type of comparison, Margulis examined what he identified as "rat fields" in relation to neighborhood sanitation in Newark, New Jersey.[23] Margulis demarcated subterranean as well as terrestrial rat fields within the city and compared complaints of rats to neighborhood sanitation. Many indicators of urban deterioration have been used in detailed analyses of health in relation to urban change. In fact, the medical geographer working on urban health problems is faced with a variety of choices in terms of selection of indicator variables as well as the kinds of health data for possible study.

Aspects of the environment in relation to housing and health are by no means new concepts, as is indicated in an historical survey developed by Martin in 1967.[24] Martin reviewed literature accumulating over approximately a century pertaining to the urban environment and health problems in England and Wales. Utilizing reconstructed historical data, Martin then performed simple pairwise correlations of indicator variables for health and housing. Martin concluded that indeed some of the contentions of such early writers as Booth and Rowntree can be statistically tested and show significance. However, Martin indicated that while these earlier generalities appear to hold true, the more recent statistical testing indicates significance, they might not be strongly correlated. For example, many writers have indicated that replacement of inhabitants of slum and near-slum areas to better (usually public) housing should lead to improved health conditions. Martin contends that this may not always be the case, and in many instances families moved from older, deteriorating neighborhoods to newer housing (estates) sometimes have not actually manifested improved health conditions. This may not be so true in other countries, and Martin indicates how some studies in the United States have indicated that health conditions have improved with relocations of families due to urban renewal.

In a 1971 geographical study of mortality of a British urban area, Griffiths expressed doubts that relocation can change health status within one generation particularly.[25] Griffiths used standardized mortality rates in the settlement of Exeter for the period 1958 to 1964 to show that in spite of a more favorable environment than found in some other parts of the United Kingdom, the social structure of Exeter is still stratified in such a manner that it is possible to identify variable health status levels in accordance with social classes. The classes are primarily determined on the basis of occupation. Griffiths used chi-square testing and Kendall's rank in a nonparametric examination of different mortality levels in relation to social class. In addition, geographic differences were identified utilizing wards of the city as units of observation. In general, Griffiths discovered that in spite of much less manufacturing activity than many other British settlements, significant health status differences exist from one ward of Exeter to another. Part of this difference was attributed to housing conditions as well as social class.

Dever's research pertaining to geographical aspects of leukemia in Buffalo and Atlanta also devoted attention to housing.[26] However, he also explained that the use of selected socioeconomic variables in statistical testing is a more refined methodology in the analysis of urban disease problems. In his study testing the contagion hypothesis of leukemia in relation to housing in Buffalo, Dever explained how different geographical scales of analysis can be expected to result in different explanations of disease variables, and this includes levels of statistical significance. Given the fact that leukemia is a low-incidence disease and may have many causes, it is extremely difficult to identify explanatory variables in associative analyses, as Dever was quick to demonstrate. In his Buffalo study he found that variables suggesting higher socioeconomic status, e.g., a high ratio of rooms per household person (and the presence of fireplaces) may be indicators of higher rates of leukemia. On the other hand, these findings may be statistical artifacts. In his exposition of leukemia in Atlanta, testing the viral etiology hypothesis, Dever used pairwise and multiple linear regression techniques employing selected socioeconomic variables indicated previously as indicators of leukemia. In both of these analyses Dever's findings were essentially negative to the extent that no clear-cut combinations of variables assisted in explaining leukemia in a manner similar to the statistical "fits" obtained when viewing mortality data for heart disease, stroke, and other leading causes of death. Dever's studies are of interest because they offer excellent methodological alternatives to the medical geographer especially concerned with low-incidence diseases in urban areas. The studies of Dever, as well as those of Martin, Griffiths, and others, lead to the general issue of explaining spatial variations in disease patterns within the context of urban ecological structure.

ASSOCIATIONS UTILIZING URBAN ECOLOGICAL STRUCTURE

As previously mentioned, published epidemiological research offers a plethora of examples of sampling selected populations and testing for significant associations with disease. The excessive use of nonparametrics can lead to the use of such tools as chi-square testing with increasingly larger samples, mostly to determine whether or not distributions are normal. As samples approach actual populations it is increasingly possible to employ more rigorous parametric tests. Examples discussed already in this chapter include linear pairwise and multiple regression. Many investigators prefer more sophisticated curvilinear statistical testing. In medical geography there has been a tendency to employ linear and curvilinear hypotheses. Since the existing literature pertaining to urban structure has utilized similar methods in the evolutionary development of associative studies, it is logical to expect examinations of human health problems within the urban ecological context.

Excellent summaries of prevailing theories on urban ecological structure are available in contributions by Berry and Rees.[27] Essentially an outgrowth of the "Chicago school" of urban analysis, the literature which has grown this century pertaining to ecological structure has its origin in the contributions of Burgess, Park, Hoyt, and later Shevkey and Bell. Burgess's early notions pertaining to the residential structure of cities, now well known, transferred biological theories into notions of competition for space followed by successions of various groups of individuals in turn leading to changing dominance of particular neighborhoods. As cities grow outward historically neighborhood social structure tends to be formed in identifiable but changing concentric rings. The ideas of Hoyt, primarily a land economist, initially indicated that high-grade residential neighborhoods do change over time and that ultimately within a city alternating sectors of high, middle and low income neighborhoods can be found. By the 1950s it became apparent, primarily because of contributions of Shevkey, Bell, and other sociologists, that both concentric and sectoral patterns of life cycle and socioeconomic status could be identified simultaneously. Work later developed at the University of Chicago under the auspices of Brian Berry offered many examples of concentric life cycle distinctions within cities, sectoral socioeconomic status distinctions and definite patterns of minority segregation, the latter often independent of the first two indicators.[28]

Utilizing these measures central to social area analysis and urban ecological structure, Girt was able to find definite associations between chronic bronchitis variations and a combination of concentric and sectoral zones in Leeds.[29] Girt first sampled the prevalence of simple chronic bronchitis within the city. He then successfully isolated general associations of bronchitis in relation to both socioeconomic status and life cycle groups. With this general descriptive backdrop, Girt further examined bronchitis utilizing environmental and behavioral variables and tested associations by calibrating a regression model. Girt's research reaffirmed the hypothesis that there are certain kinds of diseases which will correlate highly with lower income (social class) groups as well as with certain kinds of occupations. Of equal importance, there are behavioral attributes of individuals, cigarette smoking and bronchitis, for example, that can be explained via a regression analysis but demonstrate no strong spatial pattern.

In the same vein, a factor analytic approach to understanding disease distributions within Chicago was accomplished in 1968.[30] In that effort, 18 disease variables along with population density were studied for 76 generalized community areas of the city. Table 5 shows the orthogonally rotated factor matrix solution that resulted. Health measures that are generally associated with poverty conditions showed up as the first factor with nearly 40% of the variance. When scores from this factor were mapped (see Figure 81) an ecological patterning of socioeconomic status showed up in a fashion very similar to the socioeconomic status patternings reported by Rees. A second factor showing combined variance for three childhood diseases, mumps, whooping cough, and chickenpox, along with population density, gave some indication of a density combination which may have been operating within the city (Figure 82). The latter association is important because all too often different kinds of measures of "urban density" are included in associative analyses as *a priori*

Table 5. Rotated Factor Matrix Loadings for Health Measures in Chicago

Variable	Factors					Communality
	I	II	III	IV	V	
Gonorrhea	0.851	−0.350	0.271	−0.080	−0.063	0.931
Illegitimate births	0.837	−0.168	0.121	−0.095	0.077	0.758
Diarrhea	0.815	−0.015	−0.106	0.284	0.189	0.793
Premature births	0.771	−0.316	0.093	0.118	0.070	0.722
Syphilis	0.702	−0.289	0.496	−0.087	0.119	0.844
Measles	0.692	−0.485	0.154	0.205	0.077	0.785
Poisonings	0.686	−0.402	0.026	0.177	0.149	0.687
Tuberculosis	0.651	−0.350	0.258	−0.284	0.271	0.767
Infant deaths	0.537	−0.201	0.241	0.408	−0.315	0.653
Mumps	0.320	−0.810	0.038	−0.011	0.196	0.799
Population density	0.384	−0.731	0.197	0.199	−0.194	0.797
Whooping cough	0.245	−0.628	−0.143	0.286	0.178	0.588
Chickenpox	0.247	−0.532	0.155	0.103	0.468	0.598
Rheumatic fever	0.042	0.168	0.875	0.058	0.272	0.874
Scarlet fever	0.283	−0.460	0.550	0.087	−0.036	0.603
Pneumonia	0.496	−0.337	0.519	−0.166	−0.044	0.657
Rubella	0.113	−0.037	0.066	0.797	−0.073	0.660
Congenital malformation	−0.075	−0.226	0.095	0.764	0.183	0.683
Infectious hepatitis	0.151	−0.131	0.165	0.040	0.868	0.823
Percent variance	39.8	22.7	14.0	13.1	10.4	

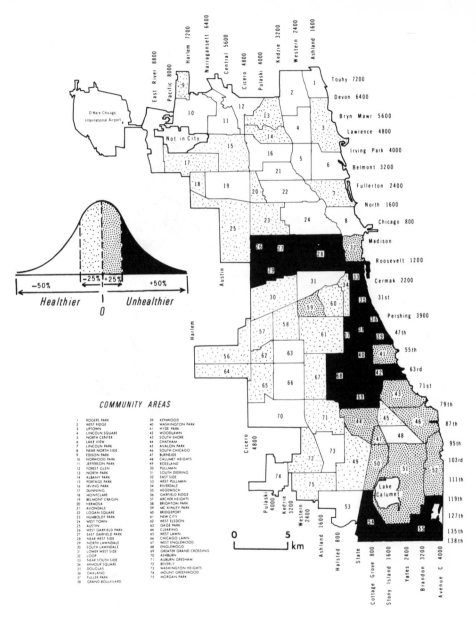

FACTOR I: THE POVERTY SYNDROME

Fig. 81. The distribution of scores representing poverty-related diseases in Chicago during the mid-1960s.

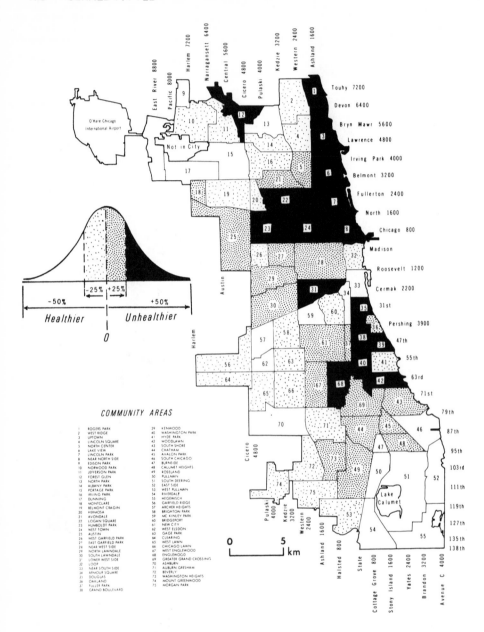

COMMUNITY AREAS

1 ROGERS PARK	39 KENWOOD
2 WEST RIDGE	40 WASHINGTON PARK
3 UPTOWN	41 HYDE PARK
4 LINCOLN SQUARE	42 WOODLAWN
5 NORTH CENTER	43 SOUTH SHORE
6 LAKE VIEW	44 CHATHAM
7 LINCOLN PARK	45 AVALON PARK
8 NEAR NORTH SIDE	46 SOUTH CHICAGO
9 EDISON PARK	47 BURNSIDE
10 NORWOOD PARK	48 CALUMET HEIGHTS
11 JEFFERSON PARK	49 ROSELAND
12 FOREST GLEN	50 PULLMAN
13 NORTH PARK	51 SOUTH DEERING
14 ALBANY PARK	52 EAST SIDE
15 PORTAGE PARK	53 WEST PULLMAN
16 IRVING PARK	54 RIVERDALE
17 DUNNING	55 HEGEWISCH
18 MONTCLARE	56 GARFIELD RIDGE
19 BELMONT CRAGIN	57 ARCHER HEIGHTS
20 HERMOSA	58 BRIGHTON PARK
21 AVONDALE	59 MC KINLEY PARK
22 LOGAN SQUARE	60 BRIDGEPORT
23 HUMBOLDT PARK	61 NEW CITY
24 WEST TOWN	62 WEST ELSDON
25 AUSTIN	63 GAGE PARK
26 WEST GARFIELD PARK	64 CLEARING
27 EAST GARFIELD PARK	65 WEST LAWN
28 NEAR WEST SIDE	66 CHICAGO LAWN
29 NORTH LAWNDALE	67 WEST ENGLEWOOD
30 SOUTH LAWNDALE	68 ENGLEWOOD
31 LOWER WEST SIDE	69 GREATER GRAND CROSSING
32 LOOP	70 ASHBURN
33 NEAR SOUTH SIDE	71 AUBURN GRESHAM
34 ARMOUR SQUARE	72 BEVERLY
35 DOUGLAS	73 WASHINGTON HEIGHTS
36 OAKLAND	74 MOUNT GREENWOOD
37 FULLER PARK	75 MORGAN PARK
38 GRAND BOULEVARD	

FACTOR II: THE DENSITY SYNDROME

Fig. 82. The distribution of scores representing density-related diseases in Chicago in the mid-1960s.

variables expected to explain major disease distributions. In the Chicago study this was not the case, and density was primarily associated with the three infectious diseases mentioned. The two primary factors are also examples of independent dimensionality in disease distributions. Subsequent testing of some of these disease measures with regression and path analysis demonstrated that selected indicator variables can be modeled to help explain the variance that individual diseases account for spatially.[31]

A word of caution is in order. While population density did cluster within the second dimension in the Chicago factor analysis, there is no guarantee if disease variables and selected indicator variables are combined in the same factor analysis that explanation of spatial variations of the diseases will be adequately achieved. The researcher stands the risk of obtaining independent dimensionality of either disease variables or particular indicators. This possibility is one of the major problems associated with the use of conventional principal components or principal axis factor analysis in associative studies.

Fortunately, canonical analysis offers a viable alternative in the process of spatial modeling for associative occurrences. While factor analysis alone is extremely useful in determining independent dimensionality of either dependent or independent sets of variables, canonical factor analysis takes two sets of variables into account. One of these sets, perhaps a matrix of disease data, can be considered the dependent or criterion variables. The second set, probably a matrix of socioeconomic and demographic variables, is considered the independent or predictor group. The two sets of variables are combined into a multivariate procedure that determines groups of dependent variables statistically associated with groups of independent variables. In the area of medical geography, the method was used in a 1974 contribution of disease associations in the Akron, Ohio area by Pyle and Lauer,[32] and more recently Briggs and Leonard used a canonical approach to mortality and ecological structure for the Houston, Texas area.[33] In both analyses, sets of disease groups had strong associations with indicators of a poverty syndrome in health status.

While the use of canonical factor analysis is a definite improvement over combining sets of dependent and independent variables in a conventional factor analysis, it still may best be viewed as an intermediate step in the associative modeling process. Although the results of a factor analysis may lead to further testing with stepwise multiple or forms of optimal regression, there are sufficient chance factors that may be encountered to call for extremely careful variable selection. Ideally, the results of a canonical factor analysis can subsequently be utilized in the process of selecting specific sets of multiple stepwise regressions for further explanation. By initially going through this form of data reduction process, the medical geographer is able to structure regressions in a more formal and meaningful manner than might be accomplished by simply collecting sets of independent and dependent variables and regressing on all possible permutations and combinations. Furthermore, a regression-path analysis can be structured in such a manner as to account for spurious associations and other possible forms of colinearity.

Now gaining acceptance and more widespread use in the epidemiological

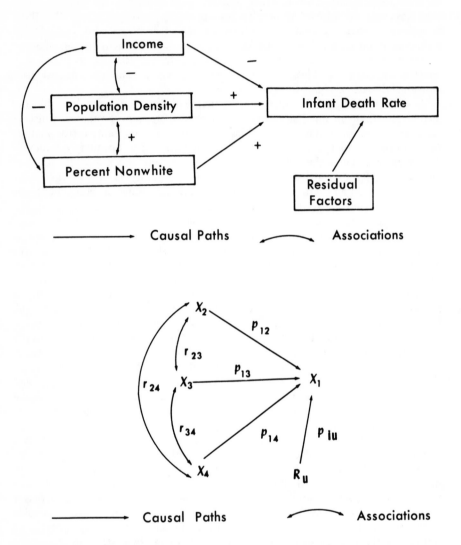

Fig. 83. The overall path analysis model generalized and how it might be used in the process of explaining associative occurrences in Infant Mortality. The above example was formulated in Chicago in the mid-1960s.

literature, path analysis has been utilized for several decades by social science researchers as a method of fully understanding regression relationships.[34] Figure 83 (bottom) shows a simple path diagram based on a multiple regression. One method of notation for this procedure is to use $P_{12}P_{13}$, etc., as path coefficients, X_1 as the dependent variable, X_2, X_3, etc., as independent variables and R_U explanatory variables not accounted for in the model. Path coefficients are standardized β coefficients which must be read back from X_1 so that $P_{12} = \beta_{12.34}$, $P_{13} = \beta_{13.24}$, etc. Causal paths are indicated by straight lines, and pairwise correlations between independent variables by curved lines (r_{23}, r_{24}, r_{34}). The results of this diagramming procedure allow the researcher to develop a better understanding of variable associations than gleaned from numerical examination alone. Using the Chicago infant mortality rate (Figure 83, top) pairwise and multiple paths were developed with family income, population density and nonwhite population as independent variables. Note the negative associations among infant mortality, density, and income. However the direct path between infant mortality and density is positive. Density and percent nonwhite show a positive pairwise correlation, and the path for percent nonwhite and infant mortality is positive. The model actually accounted for only 40% of the variance. Such results may also be used to question favored theories, for example the effects of urban population density on human health.

The results of the Chicago factor analysis (Table 5) did indicate that population density has a stronger relationship with some contagious diseases than the poverty-health syndrome indicators. Utilizing the same independent variables (income, density, and nonwhite), measles was selected as a dependent variable to be explained in a stepwise multiple regression. A simplified path analysis of the results is shown within Figure 84. The first step indicated that the strongest spatial-statistical relationship was with income, accounting for almost half of the variance. The association is negative, as indicated by the −0.688 coefficient measuring the single path. Population density entered at the second step and percent nonwhite at the third; these three variables accounted for 60% of the variance. Note that the coefficients change with the entry of each new variable. There are also unexplained residual effects with each step. This measles "explanatory model" is only one of many possible associations that can be tested, and it was used here only as an illustrative example to introduce the reader to this approach. A more sophisticated path analysis is explored later in this chapter.

In general, the researcher with sufficient information pertaining to disease distributions and hypothesized sets of associated variables will in many instances desire to rely on the results of a regression analysis in the final stages of modeling statistical explanation. Other multivariate techniques prove to be extremely useful in the modeling process when used prior to a regression because they offer the researcher certain alternative decisions in structuring final regressions. This not only saves time, but helps in accounting for problems of colinearity inherent to multivariate analysis. The following modeling framework is one sequential methodology for approaching associative analyses in such a manner.

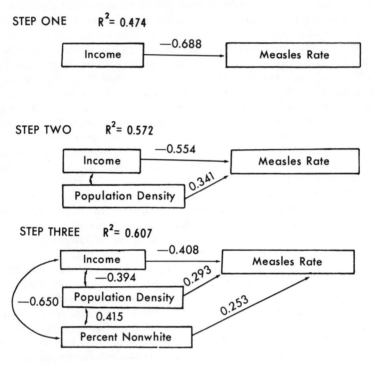

Path diagrams for three steps in regression using measles
as a dependent variable

STEP ONE $R^2 = 0.474$

STEP TWO $R^2 = 0.572$

STEP THREE $R^2 = 0.607$

Fig. 84. A step-by-step explanation of Measles in relation to income, population density and percent of the population nonwhite.

A SUGGESTED MODELING SEQUENCE

Leading causes of death in Ohio, with emphasis on heart disease and cancer, are used as the data base for a suggested modeling sequence to test associations. An issue central to this discussion, and in structuring any sort of hypothesis testing, is whether or not significant associations can be found between and among leading causes of death and selected indicators. For purposes of descriptive comparison, information pertaining to various forms of heart disease and cancer mortality for the 88 counties of the state of Ohio for the years 1965, 1970, and 1975 have been selected. Crude rates per 1,000 population have been utilized because the medical geographer often is restricted by lack of availability of more refined data. The Ohio county mortality data offer an example of deaths in counties ranging from quite sparsely populated and rural to highly urbanized. In the past some investigators have found that heart disease and cancer mortality rates are very high in rural areas while others indicate equal problems in central cities. Earlier findings in the Chicago metropolitan region, ranging from dense central city to the rural periphery, indicated that highly urbanized as well as extremely rural locations both suffer from higher than average rates of mortality for these chronic and degenerative diseases.[35] Figure 85 shows the general settlement pattern within the state in relation to population potential.[36] The northeast is highly urbanized, and heavy settlement extends along the fringes of Lake Erie. There is also a southwest to northeast axis of urban development within the state. The southeastern part of the state is generally rural in character and considered to be an extension of the Appalachian region to the southeast.

Start with Careful Examination

It is useful in any statistical analysis of disease distributions to initially gain some understanding of the data through use of descriptive measures. Table 6 contains univariate descriptive statistics for heart disease and cancer mortality (crude rates) for the three time periods. Some appreciation for differences can be obtained by realizing that for heart disease the mean rate was 657 in 1965, 723 in 1970, and 638 in 1975. The standard deviations for heart disease rates during the same times included 92.6 in 1965 to 102.4 in 1970, and 86.4 in 1975. By comparison, overall cancer rates were consistently lower. The mean in 1965 for cancer was 153; this changed to 163 in 1970 and increased to 178 in 1975. Within the context of temporal trends, it can be stated that heart disease mortality increased from 1965 to 1970 and subsequently decreased in 1975. Conversely, the overall cancer mortality rate gradually increased from one five-year period to the next.

While a wide variety of techniques are available to determine the significance of distributions, it is common practice in many health-related studies to use a chi-square structure in testing a null hypothesis that distributions are normal. Figure 86 contains histograms for each of the six distributions utilizing Sturgis' rule to determine class intervals. A chi-square value of 11.070 with 5 degrees of freedom is required as a minimum measure for conventionally accepted levels of significance. The chi-square values derived for each of the six distributions indicated that only the 1965 cancer distribution can be considered not normally distributed using this measure. In other words, for all of the other five distributions the null hypothesis must be accepted. Does this imply that the researcher should go no further? No. It is common for geographic data to be skewed.

Move to Pairwise Comparisons

Another occurrence the medical geographer embarking upon such studies should be aware of is a lack of regularity in distributions over time with spatial data. The examination of even the simplest of descriptive statistics and

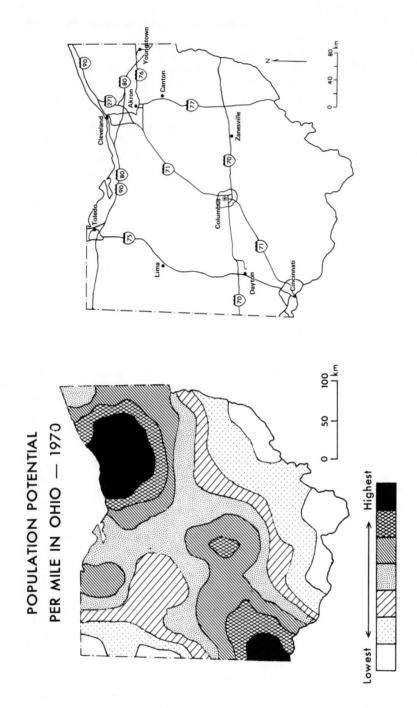

Fig. 85. Population potential per mile in Ohio in relation to major highways and cities.

Table 6. Descriptive Statistics for Heart Disease and Cancer in Ohio in 1965, 1970, and 1975[a]

Heart disease		Cancer	
		1965	
Maximum	656.5	Maximum	286.2
Minimum	211.5	Minimum	87.5
Range	445	Range	198.7
Mean	414.740	Mean	152.770
Variance	8581.770	Variance	1180.810
Standard deviation	92.640	Standard deviation	34.363
Mean deviation	72.840	Mean deviation	26.439
Median	413.6	Median	147.5
Mode	414.1	Mode	120.6/146.6/155.9/174.6
Class interval	75	Class interval	35
		1970	
Maximum	722.7	Maximum	249.5
Minimum	202.3	Minimum	96.8
Range	520.4	Range	152.7
Mean	408.774	Mean	163.805
Variance	10479.850	Variance	1128.413
Standard deviation	102.371	Standard deviation	33.592
Mean deviation	78.624	Mean deviation	25.646
Median	396.9	Median	158.9
Mode	332.9	Mode	147.2/151.6/151.9/158.9/118.5
Class interval	90	Class interval	30
		1975	
Maximum	638.4	Maximum	270.6
Minimum	197.5	Minimum	105.1
Range	440.9	Range	165.5
Mean	393.402	Mean	177.914
Variance	7467.897	Variance	1261.879
Standard deviation	86.417	Standard deviation	35.523
Mean deviation	68.521	Mean deviation	27.482
Median	379.8	Median	177.95
Mode	368.7/387.2/389.2	Mode	161.5/183.1
Class interval	75	Class interval	30

[a]88 counties.

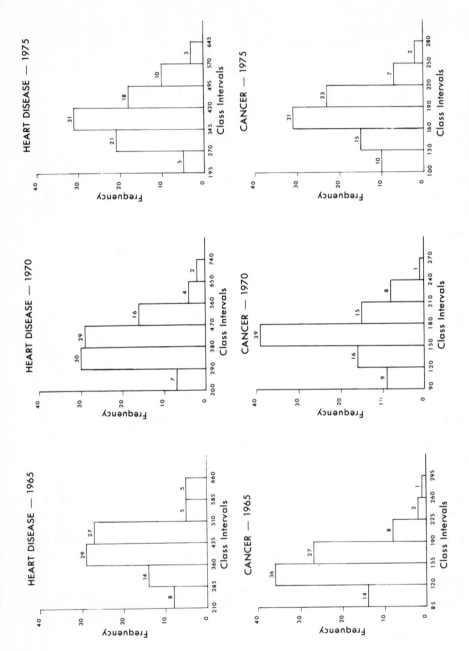

Fig. 86. Numerical distributions of Heart Disease and Cancer in Ohio from 1965 to 1970.

significance testing for the Ohio heart disease and cancer data serves as an excellent example. The next step is to find out how much variation over time exists. One method for testing distributions over time is simple linear regression. When heart disease rates for 1965 are compared in this manner with rates for the 88 counties for 1975, an R^2 value of .749 results with significance at the .01 level (see Figure 87). Such testing gives some indication that while the heart disease distributions for the two time periods may not be normally distributed, they show statistically strong and significant distributions over the ten-year time period. When the residuals or total unexplained variation from the regression are mapped, the pattern shown in Figure 88 results. The more heavily shaded areas are those parts of the state where the 1975 heart disease distributions are even higher than would be expected by the functional relationship developed using the

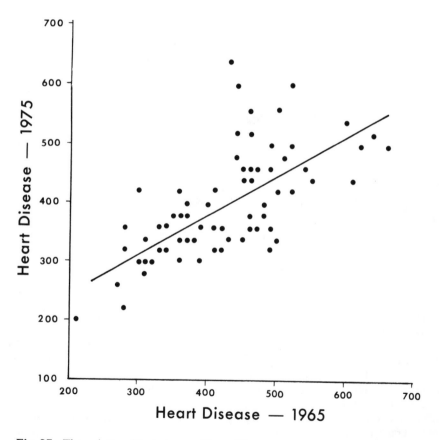

Fig. 87. The relationship between Heart Disease in 1965 and 1975 in Ohio.

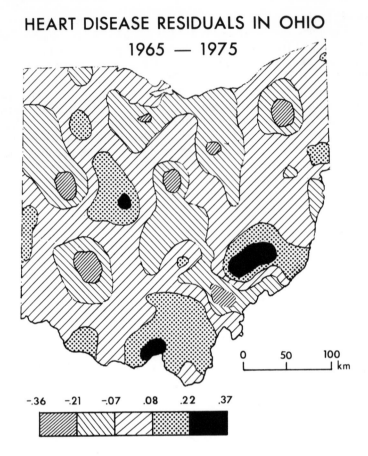

HEART DISEASE RESIDUALS IN OHIO
1965 — 1975

-.36   -.21   -.07   .08   .22   .37

Fig. 88. Residuals from the Heart Disease regression.

1965 information as an independent variable. Also, the heaviest concentrations of highest residuals are to be found in more rural southeastern parts of the state.

Similar testing for cancer distributions shows a lower multiple R^2 value (.532) significant only at the 0.5 level (see Figure 89). More temporal variance is unaccounted for with the cancer reporting. Part of the difference is that the 1965 distribution was less normal than in 1975 (according to the chi-square test). Figure 90 contains the spatial distribution of this unexplained variance. The map shows heaviest concentrations of highest or more than expected residuals in the most rural parts of the state. In other words, in addition to the rural southeast, many farming areas in the northwestern part of the state have also been

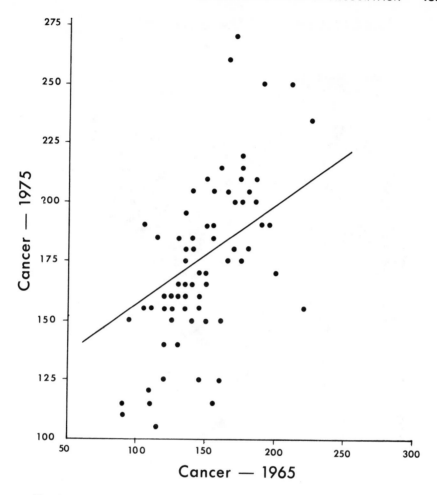

Fig. 89. The relationship between Cancer in 1965 and 1975 in Ohio.

included. A visual comparison with population potential in Ohio indicates an association which appears to be inversely related to the differences in cancer distributions (see Figure 85).

As a next step it is useful to examine various kinds of cancer and heart disease along with other leading causes of death with multivariate methods.[37] Once again, factor analysis is a useful descriptive tool in such comparisons. Since a matrix of pairwise correlations is required in the beginning steps of factor analysis, examination of this kind of information allows the medical geographer

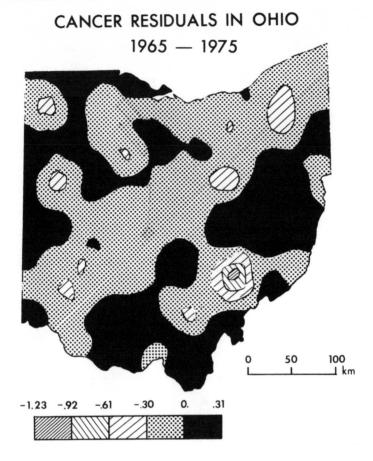

CANCER RESIDUALS IN OHIO
1965 — 1975

0   50   100
⊢——————⊣ km

−1.23   −.92   −.61   −.30   0.   .31

Fig. 90. Residuals from the Cancer regression.

to develop some initial impressions of the associations among different kinds of disease distributions. Table 7 consists of a matrix of pairwise correlations for several categorical groups of cancer and heart disease along with diabetes, influenza, stroke, and bronchitis. All correlations above or below ± .300 have been removed for clarity.

It is of interest that the intercorrelations among the various type of heart disease range from extremely high: for example, .965 when comparing ischemic heart disease with general heart disease; .937 between cardiovascular disease and heart disease; and .488 between heart disease in general and cerebrovascular disease. Similarly, the various cancer types show fairly strong to more moderate correlations. A correlation coefficient of .682 results between digestive cancer

Table 7. Pairwise Correlations of Leading Causes of Death Reported in Ohio in 1970

Disease	(1)	(2)	(3)	(4)	(5)	(6)	(7)	(8)	(9)	(10)	(11)	(12)	(13)	(14)
Malignant neoplasms (1)	1.000	0.682	0.619	0.603	0.426	–	0.637	0.387	0.608	0.580	0.597	0.363	0.517	0.371
Digestive cancer (2)	0.682	1.000	–	–	–	–	–	–	0.747	0.426	0.394	0.306	0.415	–
Respiratory cancer (3)	0.619	–	1.000	–	–	–	–	0.346	0.456	0.487	0.483	–	–	0.414
Genital cancer (4)	0.603	0.303	–	1.000	0.360	–	–	–	0.409	0.407	0.431	–	0.448	–
Urinary cancer (5)	0.426	–	–	0.360	1.000	–	–	–	–	–	–	–	–	–
Leukemia (6)	–	–	–	–	–	1.000	–	–	–	–	–	–	–	–
Other cancer (7)	0.637	–	–	–	–	–	1.000	–	–	–	–	–	–	–
Diabetes (8)	0.387	–	0.346	–	–	–	–	1.000	0.493	0.470	0.446	0.305	–	–
Cardiovascular disease (9)	0.608	0.474	0.456	0.409	–	–	–	0.493	1.000	0.937	0.901	0.717	0.538	0.405
Heart disease (10)	0.580	0.426	0.487	0.407	–	–	–	0.470	0.937	1.000	0.966	0.488	0.499	0.410
Ischemic heart disease (11)	0.597	0.394	0.483	0.431	–	–	–	0.446	0.901	0.966	1.000	0.469	0.502	0.420
Cerebrovascular disease (12)	0.363	0.306	–	–	–	–	–	0.305	0.717	0.488	0.469	1.000	0.439	–
Influenza/pneumonia (13)	0.517	0.415	–	0.448	–	–	–	–	0.538	0.499	0.502	0.439	1.000	–
Bronchitis (14)	0.371	–	0.414	–	–	–	–	–	0.405	0.410	0.420	–	–	1.000

and general malignant neoplasms, and a similar measure of .618 when comparing respiratory cancer with overall cancer. One important exception with the cancer types is leukemia. There are no correlations above ± .300 when comparing leukemia to any of the other diseases. This aspect is of particular interest in light of Dever's findings mentioned earlier. The various heart disease types show good to moderate correlations with malignant neoplasms, and most of the cancer groups have moderate to fair correlations with the heart disease variables. Examination of the correlation matrix serves as a preview to the multivariate statistical associations uncovered after the subsequent factoring process.

Explore with Factor Analysis

The correlation matrix also serves as an input to the principal axis factor analysis utilized here and recommended for similar studies. After orthogonal rotation, four "independent" factors emerged. Factor loadings are contained within Table 8. The first and most important factor to emerge consists of the heart disease group along with influenza and pneumonia. This factor accounts for more than 65% of the total variance and can be described as a clustering of major heart disease mortality. When scores for all the factors are mapped (Figure 91), four different spatial distributions result. Initial interpretation of the factor

Table 8. Rotated Factor Matrix Loadings of Ohio Mortality, 1970

Variable	Factors				Communality
	I	II	III	IV	
Diabetes	0.372	0.284	0.089	0.170	0.256
Cardiovascular disease	0.909	0.295	0.136	0.208	0.977
Heart disease	0.822	0.392	0.046	0.315	0.930
Ischemic heart disease	0.775	0.399	0.589	0.372	0.902
Cerebrovascular disease	0.733	0.015	0.161	−0.065	0.567
Influenza/pneumonia	0.502	0.082	0.352	0.130	0.399
Respiratory cancer	0.231	0.829	0.143	0.042	0.763
Bronchitis/emphysema/asthma	0.278	0.453	0.200	−0.073	0.328
Malignant neoplasms	0.338	0.434	0.740	0.375	0.991
Digestive cancer	0.464	−0.015	0.703	−0.101	0.720
Other cancer	−0.083	0.372	0.650	0.109	0.581
Genital cancer	0.290	−0.044	0.423	0.601	0.627
Urinary cancer	0.051	0.138	0.261	0.441	0.284
Leukemia	0.084	−0.031	−0.107	0.542	0.314
Percent of variance	65.5	14.9	10.4	9.2	

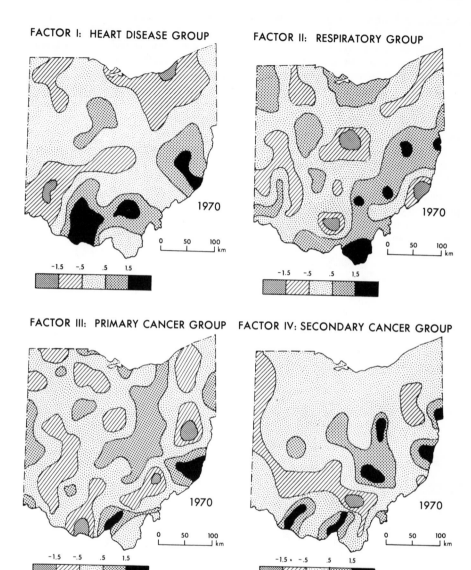

Fig. 91. Distributions of scores for four factors representing leading causes of death in Ohio in 1970.

one map indicates the highest concentrations are in the rural southeastern part of the state for these combined heart disease-related variables. Since much of the literature indicates that heart disease is a problem in urban as well as rural areas, regression testing can be useful to help explain the factor one score pattern. Factor scores were weighted to remove negative values and regressed against population potential. The best fit proved to be the negative second degree polynomial relationship shown within Figure 92. The parts of the state with lowest population potential, not unexpectedly, reflect high disease scores and low population potential. Many of these areas are rural-farm with low incomes and older populations. However, some parts of the state with higher population potential also have higher rates than those in the intermediate range. These are the most metropolitan areas. A dual relationship was identified by the curvilinear fit results in a reverse "J-curve" with an R^2 value of .524. In this instance it is possible to account for nearly half of the pairwise variance.

The second factor, accounting for nearly 15% of the multivariate variance, is a combination of respiratory cancer and other forms of respiratory disease. Scores

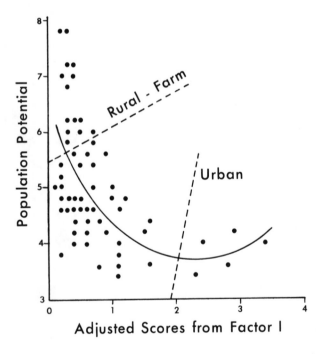

Fig. 92. The curvilinear relationship between adjusted scores from the first factor (see Figure 91) and population potential.

for this respiratory syndrome are mapped within Figure 91 also. Since the second factor is independent of the first, the correlation with population potential is low. The distribution of high scores incorporates large areas of the southeastern part of the state. The respiratory group pattern raises the question of possible future testing with information pertaining to man-made environmental hazards, but the implication of age associations is also present. In addition, future research might include the testing of associations with behavioral variables at the microscale level.

The third factor can be considered a primary cancer group. Malignant neoplasms and several cancer types account for approximately 10% of the variance. Remembering that some of the cancer distributions do not appear to be as spatially consistent over time as the heart disease group, the most useful comparison of distributions of factor scores for the third factor is with scores mapped from the fourth factor consisting of genital cancer, urinary cancer, and leukemia (a secondary cancer group). Since these two factors are independent of one another and the patterns on the two maps are different, it is difficult to make broad sweeping statements about the distribution of *all* cancer in Ohio. Many different explanatory variables should be used to gain some explanation of these patterns.

This demonstration in the use of factor analysis should be considered an intermediate step used to uncover independent multivariate dimensions. Some of the problems that can result in utilizing the results of a factor analysis as an end result in the research process should be understood. In this exercise the factor analysis model does help explain common patterns of variation among the heart disease-related group. A respiratory cluster was uncovered. The results also contain primary and secondary cancer groups. The factor analysis adds some explanation to the differences in levels of significance when comparing cancer distributions. Since factor analysis is not a "causal" model, no hypothesized explanatory variables were included in the matrix.

Canonical Explanation

The next step is now taken by incorporating a set of independent or explanatory variables into the matrix of disease measures used for the factor analysis in an attempt to identify multivariate associations. The variables included in Table 9 as percent urban, two income extremes, several age groups, and physicians and hospital beds in relation to the population are considered a predictor set in a canonical factor analysis. As shown within Table 9, sets of pairwise correlations among disease and predictor variables vary considerably. For example, the correlation between heart disease and percent of the population over 65 years of age is .871. A negative correlation (−.615) results when comparing percent of the population 18 to 44 years of age with heart disease. Malignant neoplasms correlate well with percent of the population over 65 (.650), and with percent of the population from 45 to 64 (.582). Also, the correlation between malignant neoplasms and percent of the population 18 to 44 years of age is −.455.

Table 9. Pairwise Correlations of Dependent (Criterion) and
Independent (Predictor) Variables[a]

Disorder	Percent					
	Urban residents	18–44 years of age	45–64 years of age	Over 65 years of age	$5,000 annual income	$15,000–24,999 annual income
Malignant neoplasms	–	−0.455	0.582	0.650	0.460	−0.500
Digestive cancer	–	−0.355	0.330	0.513	0.399	−0.402
Respiratory cancer	–	–	0.492	0.447	0.386	−0.365
Genital cancer	–	−0.321	0.344	0.450	0.359	−0.416
Urinary cancer	–	–	–	–	–	–
Leukemia	–	–	–	–	–	–
Other cancer	–	–	–	–	–	–
Cardiovascular disease	−0.451	−0.607	0.649	0.890	0.799	−0.820
Heart disease	−0.393	−0.615	0.642	0.871	0.751	−0.766
Ischemic heart disease	−0.344	−0.595	0.668	0.854	0.725	−0.743
Cerebrovascular disease	−0.433	−0.368	0.425	0.591	0.579	−0.628
Influenza and pneumonia	–	−0.330	–	0.546	0.486	−0.487
Bronchitis	–	–	0.317	–	0.358	−0.369

[a]Physicians per 10,000 population—none for all disorders; Beds per 1,000 population—none for all disorders.

Since the literature on health care planning (discussed in more detail in the next chapter) places emphasis on the importance of the ratio of physicians and hospital beds to population, these two variables were added for comparative purposes. No strong pairwise correlations, i.e., more than ± .300 resulted. This does not imply significant multivariate associations might not show up in the canonical factor analysis. One of the advantages of this method is that multivariate dimensionality can be identified for weakly correlated variables. Table 10 contains the three most important dimensions resulting from the canonical factoring. The top or predictor set includes the physician and hospital independent variables.

The canonical multivariate associations add a degree of explanation beyond the previous steps in this modeling process. For example, the first canonical factor with an R^2 of .907 includes in the criterion or disease set highest loadings on the major heart disease measures as well as many of the cancer measures. Comparing these groups of high loadings with the predictor set, the age groups 45 to 64 and over 65 as well as percent of the income below $5,000 annually show the highest positive associations. This verifies known cancer and heart disease associations occuring more with increasing age and in lower income groups. Inverse or negative associations in the predictor set include percent of the

Table 10. Canonical Factor Structure Mortality in Ohio

Variable	Canonical factor loadings		
	I	II	III
Criterion set: mortality			
Malignant neoplasms	.709	.214	.539
Digestive cancer	.520	.397	.279
Respiratory cancer	.546	−.072	.458
Genital cancer	.486	.096	.240
Urinary cancer	.220	.248	.225
Leukemia	.200	.136	−.009
Other cancer	.272	.139	.314
Cardiovascular disease	.978	−.008	−.165
Heart disease	.944	.111	−.076
Ischemic heart disease	.934	.069	.039
Cerebrovascular disease	.680	−.281	−.302
Influenza/pneumonia	.549	.249	−.033
Bronchitis	.433	−.463	.172
Predictor set			
Percent urban	−.414	.082	.821
Percent 18–44 years of age	−657	−.271	.016
Percent 45–64 years of age	.736	−.147	.399
Percent over 65 years of age	.950	.253	−.088
Percent less than $5,000	.828	.005	−.315
Percent $15,000–$24,999	−.859	.091	.244
Physicians per 1,000	−.141	−.059	.698
Beds per 1,000	.154	−.014	.260
R^2	0.907	0.411	0.299
Criterion set			
Variance extracted	0.395	0.053	0.072
Redundancy	0.358	0.022	0.022
Predictor set			
Variance extracted	0.439	0.022	0.194
Redundancy	0.398	0.009	0.058

population urban, percent of the population under 18 years of age, and percent of the population with higher incomes. This result offers a dual explanation for leading causes of death. It should also be understood that the canonical factor analysis results offer overlapping explanation from one factor to another, and the various dimensions should therefore not be taken to have the degrees of independence from one to the next as assumed within factor analysis.

The third canonical factor exemplifies this possibility, with an R^2 of .299 suggesting a strong association between some of the cancer types and percent of the population urban. The ratio of physicians to population variable also has a significant loading on this factor, but this association may exist because of concentrations of more physicians in urban places (see Chapter 7).

The canonical factor analysis offers a modeling step beyond factor analysis by incorporating groups of independent and dependent variables simultaneously. From such results it is possible for the medical geographer to select and specify different sets of predictor variables to be used in stepwise multiple regressions so that the effects of several independent variables on the various disease or dependent variables can be measured in different ways. By accomplishing a canonical factor analysis first, the researcher is better able to model the next step.

Stepwise Regression: A Selection Process

While many more regressions are possible than those used as examples below, three different associations have been selected for purposes of explaining the final step in this modeling process. The first of these regressions considered on the basis of the canonical analysis is heart disease as a dependent variable. In a stepwise fashion, age of the population from 45-65, percent of the population over 65, and percent of the population with incomes less than $5,000 annually are used as dependent variables. Figure 93 includes diagrammatic information from each of the three steps. In the first step, proportion of the population over 65 years of age is entered into the model and accounts for almost 76% of the variance, thus indicating a high degree of explanation initially. In the second step, 78% of the variance is explained with the addition of the low income variable. The third and final step, that considering all three independent variables simultaneously, includes 80% of the variance. These three variables can be defined as key indicators measuring degrees of statistical explanation of heart disease mortality within the state by county. However, it should be noted from the pairwise correlations and the canonical factoring that all of these associations are positive.

There are also negative associations with heart disease that could be considered. While three variables, percent of the population urban, percent of the population under 18 years of age, and that indicting a higher income group, might have been added with the above model, little more of the variance would have been explained. By separating canonical associations and following the same modeling process an alternate explanation to heart disease can be offered. In the first step (see Figure 94) percent of the population earning more than $15,000

MODEL ONE   R² = .759

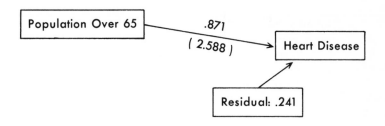

MODEL TWO   R² = .782

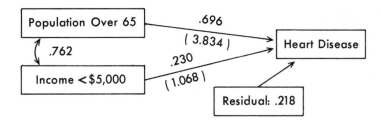

MODEL THREE   R² = .807

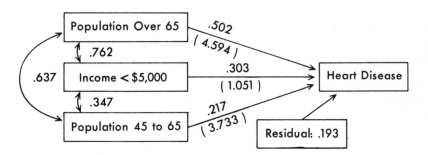

Fig. 93. The stepwise process of explaining Heart Disease mortality in Ohio using path analysis.

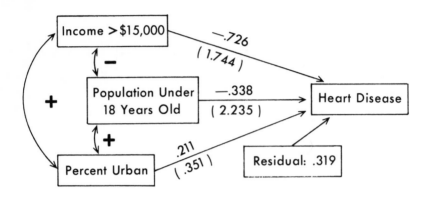

$$R^2 = .681$$

Fig. 94. An alternative model for Heart Disease in Ohio using path analysis.

annually is entered as a variable and accounts for 58% of the variance; however, this is an inverse relationship. In the second step, 65% of the variance can be accounted for by adding the variable indicating a higher proportion of more youthful populations. In the third step, not quite two percent more variance is added by including the variable percent urban. This alternative explanatory model explains 68% of the variance by the end of the third step. The two regression models utilized not only support the earlier "reverse J" association explained when regressing adjusted factor scores against population potential, they also offer specific measured associations from two different sets of independent variables.

Utilizing the same three variables taken as independent in the first of the heart disease regressions (percent of the population 45 to 65, percent of the population over 65, and percent of the population with annual incomes under $5,000 a year annually), a regression with malignant neoplasms as an independent variable was also accomplished. In that regression example, only two steps proved to be significant. The most important variable was percent of the population over 65 years of age, and it accounted for 65% of the variance. When the second significant variable showing percent of the population from 45 to 65 was added, a total of 68% of the variance was accounted for with these two variables. Once again, this finding is somewhat in keeping with the associations discussed earlier in this chapter.

The entire step-by-step modeling process accomplished in this chapter with the Ohio examples was not intended as a numerical exercise. Instead, it was developed as an example of modeling often necessary for associative studies in medical geography. The preponderance of nonparametric significance testing in much of the biomedical literature proves to be extremely useful when initially determining significance levels for spatially derived health data. Further nonparametric testing in many epidemiological studies is appropriately accomplished within a more clinical and quite often nonspatial context. Given basic assumptions underlying certain principles in spatial analysis, there is little doubt that parametric testing procedures ranging from simple pairwise correlations through different kinds of factor analysis to multiple regression assist in explaining distributions. In many cases the final results of such analyses do not depart drastically from findings of a more clinical nature. For example, heart disease risk with increasing age and lower income is well known. Since similar kinds of associations can be uncovered through the use of parametric tests with spatial data, the medical geographer can augment biomedical and epidemiological findings by explaining spatial similarities and differences. This is more than disease mapping, because specific associative measurement techniques are utilized. The application of the procedures recommended in this chapter have equal utility in the health care delivery planning process.

NOTES

[1] N. D. McGlashan. "Geographical Evidence on Medical Hypotheses," *Tropical and Geographical Medicine,* Vol. 19 (1967), pp. 333–343.

[2] Marvin W. Mikesell. "Geography as the Study of Environment: An Assessment of Some Old and New Commitments" in Ian R. Manners and Marvin W. Mikesell (eds.), *Perspectives on Environment.* Washington: Association of American Geographers (1974), pp. 1–23.

[3] See Chapter 2, note 9.

[4] Carol Vargo. "The Use of Data in Health Planning," unpublished Master's thesis, University of Akron, Department of Urban Studies.

[5] Seephen C. Joseph, Dieter Koch-Weser, and Ned Wallace. *Worldwide Overview of Health and Disease.* New York: Springer (1977).

[6] Fred Burbank. *Patterns of Cancer Mortality in the United States: 1959-1967.* Washington: Superintendent of Documents, National Cancer Institute Monograph 33 (1971).

[7] See Chapter 3, note 25.

[8] P. Bogovski, M. Purde, and M. Rahu. "Some Epidemiological Data on Lung Cancer in the USSR" in U. Mohr, D. Schmahl, and L. Tomatis (eds.), *Air Pollution and Cancer in Man.* Lyon: IARC Scientific Publications No. 16 (1977), pp. 241–246.

[9] G. W. Kafuko and D. P. Burkitt. "Burkitt's Lymphoma and Malaria," *International Journal of Cancer,* Vol. 6 (1970), pp. 1–9.

[10] A. M. G. Campbell. "Epidemiology of Multiple Sclerosis (A Viewpoint)," *International Journal of Environmental Studies,* Vol. 4 (1973), pp. 117–120.

[11] Edward T. Creagan and Joseph F. Fraumeni, Jr. "Cancer Mortality Among American Indians, 1950-67," *Journal of the National Cancer Institute,* Vol. 49 (1972), pp. 959–967.

[12] Bengt W. Johansson. "Myocardial Infarction in Malmo, 1960-1968," *Acta Medica Scandanavia,* Vol. 191 (1972), pp. 505–515.

[13] Nyman A. Scotch. "Sociocultural Factors in the Epidemiology of Zulu Hypertension," *American Journal of Public Health,* Vol. 53 (1963), pp. 1205–1213.

[14] Meryl H. Haber and Peter Lipkovic. "Thyroid Cancer in Hawaii," *Cancer,* Vol. 25 (1970), pp. 1224–1227.

[15] Ronald J. Kuzma, Cecilia M. Kuzma, and C. Ralph Buncher. "Ohio Drinking Water Source and Cancer Rates," *American Journal of Public Health,* Vol. 67 (1977), pp. 725–729.

[16] Eleanor J. MacDonald. "Demographic Variation in Cancer in Relation to Industrial and Environmental Influence," *Environmental Health Perspectives,* Vol. 17 (1976), pp. 153–166.

[17] Melinda S. Meade. "Community Health and Changing Hazards in a Voluntary Agricultural Resettlement," *Social Science and Medicine (Medical Geography),* Vol. 12 (1978), pp. 95–102.

[18] Masako Momiyama-Sakamoto, Juichiro Takeuchi, and Kunie Katayama. "Signs Seen in Japan of Deseasonality in Human Mortality," *Papers in Meteorology and Geophysics,* Vol. 26 (June, 1975), pp. 9–34.

[19] John M. Hunter. "The Summer Disease—Some Field Evidence on Seasonality in Childhood Lead Poisoning," *Social Science and Medicine (Medical Geography),* Vol. 12 (1978), pp. 85–94.

[20] Raphael J. Caprio, Harry L. Margulis, and Morris M. Joselow. "Lead Absorption in Children and Its Relationship to Urban Traffic Densities," *Archives of Environmental Health,* Vol. 28 (1974), pp. 195–197; and "Residential Location, Ambient Air Lead Pollution and Lead Absorption in Children," *The Professional Geographer,* Vol. 27 (1975), pp. 37–42.

[21] Harry L. Margulis. "The Control and Prevention of Pediatric Lead Poisoning in East Orange, New Jersey," *Journal of Environmental Health,* Vol. 39 (1977), pp. 362–365.

[22] Robert Lewis and Lawrence Chadzynski. "Evolutionary Changes in the Environment, Population and Health Affairs in Detroit, 1968-1971," *American Journal of Public Health,* Vol. 64 (1974), pp. 557–567.

[23] Harry L. Margulis. "Rat Fields, Neighborhood Sanitation, and Rat Complaints in Newark, New Jersey," *Geographical Review,* Vol. 67 (1977), pp. 221–231.

[24] A. E. Martin. "Environment, Housing and Health," *Urban Studies,* Vol. 4 (1967), pp. 1–21.

[25] M. Griffiths. "A Geographical Study of Mortality in an Urban Area," *Urban Studies,* Vol. 8 (1971), pp. 111–120.

[26] G. E. Alan Dever. "Leukemia in Atlanta, Georgia," *Southeastern Geographer,* Vol. 12 (1972), pp. 91–100. Also G. E. A. Dever. "Leukaemia and Housing: An Intra-Urban Analysis" in N. D. McGlashan (ed.), *Medical Geography: Techniques and Field Studies.* London: Methuen (1972), pp. 233–245.

[27] Brian J. L. Berry and Frank Horton. *Geographic Perspectives on Urban Systems.* Englewood Cliffs: Prentice-Hall (1970), Chapter 10.

[28] *Economic Geography,* Vol. 47, No. 2 (supplement) (1971).

[29] John L. Girt. "Simple Chronic Bronchitis and Urban Ecological Structure" in N. D. McGlashan (ed.), *Medical Geography: Techniques and Field Studies.* London: Methuen (1972), pp. 211–231.

[30] Gerald F. Pyle. "Some Aspects of Urban Medical Geography," unpublished Master's thesis, University of Chicago, Department of Geography (1968).

[31] Gerald F. Pyle and Philip H. Rees. "Modeling Patterns of Death and Disease in Chicago," *Economic Geography,* Vol. 47 (1971), pp. 475–488.

[32] Gerald F. Pyle and Bruce M. Lauer. "Comparing Spatial Configurations: Hospital Service Areas and Disease Rates," *Economic Geography,* Vol. 51 (1975), pp. 50–68.

[33] Ronald Briggs and William A. Leonard, IV. "Mortality and Ecological Structure: A Canonical Approach," *Social Science and Medicine (Medical Geography),* Vol. 11 (1977), pp. 757–762.

[34] M. J. Burridge, C. W. Schwabe, and T. W. Pullum. "Path Analysis: Application in an Epidemiological Study of Echinococcosis in New Zealand," *Journal of Hygiene*, Vol. 78 (1977), pp. 135–149.

[35] Gerald F. Pyle. *Heart Disease, Cancer and Stroke in Chicago: A Geographical Analysis with Facilities Plans for 1980.* Chicago: University of Chicago, Research Monograph No. 134 (1971).

[36] For an excellent explanation of the concept of population potential, see Peter J. Taylor. *Quantitative Methods in Geography: An Introduction to Spatial Analysis.* Boston: Houghton Mifflin (1977), pp. 52–58.

[37] U.S. Department of Health, Education, and Welfare, National Center for Health Statistics. *Vital Statistics of the United States, 1970,* Volume II. part B. Rockville, Maryland: DHEW (1974), pp. 7–634.

Chapter 7

GEOGRAPHICAL APPLICATIONS IN PLANNING FOR IMPROVED HEALTH CARE DELIVERY

In a recent comparison of prevailing academic research trends in medical geography, Andrew Learmonth raises the question whether there are "two medical geographies or one?"[1] Learmonth's reference is to many of the trends discussed within the first chapter of this book compared to the increasing number of published works about the geography of health care delivery systems particularly important to North American researchers. Clearly, health care delivery systems differ to varying degrees from one nation to another. Milton Roemer offers a generalized comparative typology of international health care delivery systems in a recent publication.[2] According to Roemer three factors, economic, sociopolitical, and cultural-historical, have influenced the growth and development of different health care systems. Political systems are subdivided into centralized, moderate, and localized structures while economic systems are considered to be either affluent, marginal, or very poor. Different cultures often cross national boundaries but have some influence on human behavior in seeking health care. Within this context, Roemer suggests five types of health care systems:

1. Free enterprise
2. Welfare state
3. Transitional state
4. Underdeveloped
5. Socialist state

A more or less "open market" exists in free enterprise health care systems. The country most closely approximating such a system is the United States.

Within welfare state health care systems, delivery is ideally governed by a social philosophy of egalitarianism and some form of governmental control. Examples of welfare state health care delivery systems include France, Sweden, the United Kingdom, and to some extent, Canada. In transition states, quite often countries with extractive economies, health care delivery systems are undergoing different forms of development. Within many of these countries, examples include Latin America and the Middle East, the more affluent respond to proprietary health care services. In underdeveloped states (Roemer prefers the latter term to "developing") the majority of the population is simply out of the reach of any organized health care delivery. Aside from randomly located charitable and perhaps experimental clinics, there is often little more available than the services of the traditional healer. Within Roemer's typology health care in a socialist state is entirely controlled by strong centralized government. Obvious examples of the latter include the Soviet Union and the People's Republic of China.

The use of geographical applications in planning for health care delivery varies considerably from one type of system to another. Within the Soviet Union, medical geographers are not directly involved in planning for locations of health care delivery facilities. This function is the domain of a separate centralized organization. In many European countries with government-sponsored health care delivery programs, important geographical factors are taken into consideration. Sweden is probably the best example. Since national policies and events often influence the direction of research trends, studies by medical geographers are often directed in a similar manner. In what appears to many Europeans to be a peculiar preoccupation with the geography of health care, many North American medical geographers have directed efforts toward the utilization of principles of spatial analysis to solutions of practical health care problems and applications. Furthermore, this preoccupation, if that is what it really is, has given rise to some confusion within academic circles in North America pertaining to definitions of medical geography.

If there are differences of opinion pertaining to the definition of medical geography within the discipline in North America, they become insignificant when compared to the conflict that exists in the United States relative to planning health care delivery. This conflict, deeply rooted in the free enterprise system, has for the moment become what some have termed "institutionalized."[3] The overall problem is much larger in scope than any clarification of precisely what the role of the geographer could or should actually be in planning health care delivery. The problem is the result of an ongoing interplay of special interest groups, including: major industrial interests; organized labor; an emerging hierarchy of federal, state, and local health planning authorities; insurance interests; hospitals and hospital organizations; and well-organized physician professional groups. The result is a massive quagmire consisting of continuous moves and countermoves on the part of these varied special interest groups. As we approach the latter part of the 20th century, no solution appears over the horizon. It is far too presumptuous to assume that the prudent use of geographical applications offers any panacea to the problem; however, knowledge of geographical aspects of the health care delivery system within the United States is important to developing an understanding of human health care problems.

THE IDENTIFICATION OF SPATIAL COMPONENTS

In *Health Care Delivery: Spatial Perspectives,* Shannon and Dever offer the most concise summary of geographic aspects of health care published to date.[4] In this contribution they explain many ways in which the geographer can apply his analytic skills to the identification of health care problems. Within the context of the overall organization of health care, important relationships of a geographical nature between physicians and patients lead to a broad understanding of idealized hierarchies of medical care delivery. Shannon and Dever also explain spatial patterns of health resources, including variable distributions of physicians nationally and within metropolitan areas. An important contribution of Shannon and Dever includes the impact of geographic factors on institutional policies. In fact, general policy issues pertaining to health care in the United States both influence and require the input of medical geographers.

Developmental Trends to the Mid-Twentieth Century

By the end of the Second World'War, the United States had developed a wide array of health care facilities.[5] Health care delivery mechanisms that existed by the middle of the 20th century were often described by critics as "disorganized," "unrelated," "overlapping" in terms of patterns of care. They were also considered to be "uneconomic," "ineffective," and "haphazard in development." A national commission on hospital care described the general lack of coordianted planning in the United States as generally meager in relation to the country's resources. It was thought that there was little supervision in the establishment, organization, or quality of care in many hospitals. Few states had any organized legislation pertaining to the quality of health care; this was left to established professional organizations. In general the commission propounded a need for national health care planning policies. Regardless of any possible hierarchy of health care delivery services ranging from physicians' offices through clinics to hospitals, the hospitals became an initial target for advocates of systematic national health care planning.

Any planning efforts that had developed prior to 1946 were based on hospital initiative. Degrees of planning were often determined by type of hospital control, and the implementation of plans was further determined by revenues. Three kinds of hospital had developed in accordance with type of ownership. These groups included: (1) *governmental* (federal, state, and local) facilities depending upon public funds for operating; (2) *voluntary* (community organization, church, fraternal, etc.) hospitals operating on charity and fees as sources of revenue; and (3) *proprietary* (private) units operating on profits. Between 1920 and 1946 isolated plans, either local or statewise, had been developed and there were perhaps only a half dozen of any real significance.[6] Some of these plans did lend impetus to a thrust which became the basis for post-World War Two health care delivery planning. The thrust consisted of methods whereby the adequacy of facilities serving populations could be improved and how methods of coordination among facilities might be accomplished. These two basic issues were the result of a long series of developmental trends in the United States.

European health care delivery traditions were carried to the United States during the colonial era. European needs for collective health care treatment centers were most clearly manifested as a result of the black death. When existing treatment facilities and personnel were taxed beyond all human limits, only limited choices were available. Those who could afford treatment when available, received it privately. Those who could not relied upon charity. Charity treatment, in turn, was in the hands of the church. After the Reformation pest houses developed in Protestant countries, and the church continued its function in Catholic regions. Hispanic Catholics in particular transferred the concept of the chapel-mission to the new world. In colonial North America the Protestant traditions were largely reflected. Almshouses were created in the early 18th century for public charity cases, including the sick-poor, the poverty-stricken, the orphaned, the handicapped, the mentally ill, and any other persons considered derelicts. William Penn established the first of these facilities in Philadelphia in 1713. By 1750 most of the larger urban places had almshouses. Eventually many of the long-term inhabitants of these institutions were sent to specialized asylums.

By the middle of the 18th century another trend had developed, and those who could afford to pay began to use voluntary hospitals. The first successful such venture has been attributed to the efforts and influence of Benjamin Franklin. In 1751 Franklin solicited 2,000 pounds from the Assembly of Pennsylvania with the stipulation that he would find the means to match that amount from private contributions. The result of this agreement was the Pennsylvania Hospital. The trend continued as New York Hospital was founded in 1773, Massachusetts General Hospital in 1810, and New Haven Hospital in 1826. The concept of voluntary hospitals continued, becoming the first major break from European health care delivery methods.[7] In comparison to the first part of the 20th century, the 19th century hospital growth rate was slow. However, many hospitals developed medical schools in conjunction with advances in biomedical knowledge. By 1873 there were 178 hospitals of all kinds in the United States, with a total bed capacity of a little less than 35,000.[8] One-third of these hospital beds were for mental patients in custodial care. With the advent of new medical knowledge in the latter part of the 19th century, the number of hospitals in the United States increased significantly. The death-house stigma had been removed and public demands led to unprecedented growth.

Dubbed the "free-wheeling" era of development, the period from the turn of this century to 1946 was one of rapid growth in health care delivery facilities.[9] It was at this time that the infrastructure for our present system of health care delivery facilities became firmly implanted. The voluntary short-term hospital dominated a system which was characterized nationally by uneven geographical distributions of facilities, no overall national coordination, and no major planning programs. Hospitals were largely the result of local initiative or private philanthropy. Large medical schools provided health care of the best quality in selected urban locations. The attitude in many rural areas was one of perceiving the hospital as the last possible resort. An overall lack of financial resources inhibited the construction of many hospitals and the formation of other health care plans in more remote rural locales. In 1929 the Depression marked the end of fifty years of some of the most rapid growth in hospital construction the United States had witnessed. Earlier, in 1909, the American Medical Association census indicated 4,359 hospitals.[10] By 1928 there were 6,852 hospitals; however, conditions during the Depression forced approximately 700 hospitals to close by 1938. There was little construction activity during the Depression. Government-supported hospitals were able to survive at a somewhat better rate than the other kinds. In spite of the leveling off in numbers of hospitals during this period, the number of beds available to the population gradually increased (see Figure 95). While the number of hospitals decreased 6.4% from 1927 to 1941, the number of hospital beds increased at a rate of 55.2%[11] Governmental hospital beds increased at the most rapid rate (70%). Proportions of ownership by 1945 included: voluntary hospitals with 50% of the total; governmental hospitals with 29%; and proprietary hospitals, 21%.

During the first half of this century other health care delivery facilities were also changing in orientation. Public health departments that had grown slowly prior to the First World War were on the increase in scope and numbers.[12] In 1935 there were 561 county and multicounty health departments representing approximately 760 counties, and by 1946 the number of counties covered and the quantity of departments had nearly doubled. Many had assumed substantial responsibility in taking care of the health care needs of charity patients. During the Depression, Title VI provisions of the 1935 Federal Social Security Act included health care for the medically indigent. The almshouses were being replaced.

Prior to 1946 there was indeed a lack of coordinated planning to meet health needs. Hospitals were constructed either where the land was available, near major transportation arteries, or adjacent to high income residential neighborhoods. Some interests had considered planning, and the first formal effort was accomplished by the New York Academy of Medicine in 1920. By 1927 the American Hospital Association officially recommended a ratio of five beds per thousand population for general community hospitals. The AHA suggestion was followed by many who could. In 1931 the Bingham Associate Fund made recommendations for coordinated planning in New England. The Michigan Hospital Survey Committee developed a plan in 1942 and the city of Rochester came forth with yet another in 1946. The need for planning had been clearly demonstrated, and this need was filled by the Hill–Burton Act of 1946.

Three Decades of Planning Program Development

The several decades following World War II witnessed a series of public laws enacted in the United States, mostly in the form of amendments to the Public

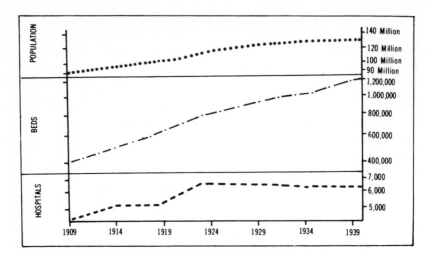

A comparison of the growth of hospitals and hospital beds,
1909 — 1939

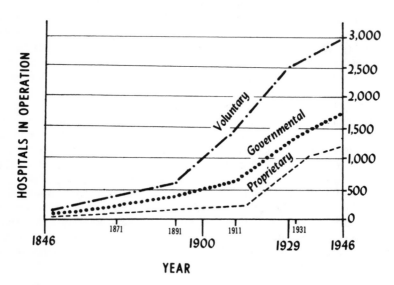

The growth of various hospitals by type of sponsorship

Fig. 95. The growth of hospitals and hospital beds in the United States
to 1939 and a comparison of different types of sponsorship.

Health Service Act, that paralleled the growth of hospitals in the country prior to the Depression. This series of program development is depicted within Figure 96 as various plateaus of growth in health care delivery planning. The Hill-Burton Act of 1946 was a landmark in health planning. Freedom from economic depression and war had allowed the United States to gather its resources and attempt to begin correcting the shortcomings of the existing system. The intent of the Hill-Burton Act was to supply aid in constructing hospitals in geographic locations most in need. As with any such program, it expanded over time. Initially, however, it was the responsibility of individual states to survey their existing supplies of hospitals to determine needs. Funds would be supplied to help in new construction after the surveys were completed. States were given federal funds on a per capita income basis through planning agencies they had established. States first had to establish plans, and in order to establish these plans some information pertaining to travel habits of hospital patients was required. This was one of the first clearcut needs documented requiring geographic data as information required. Hill-Burton programs lasted for approximately two decades. During that time much had been accomplished.[13] Systematic statewide planning of hospital facilities had begun. Standards of need were established. A better distribution of facilities resulted. Improvements were noted in hospital design and operation. Effective cooperation between governmental units and preexisting voluntary health care agencies resulted, and medical care in some low income states and rural parts of the country was improved.

Improvements in handling and the increased expansion of scope over time of Hill-Burton programs led to increased amounts of social capital both from private and public sorces as inputs into the hospital system. In addition, amendments to the Hill-Burton Act were increasingly geared toward a metropolitan society. The natural outcome of these changes was the establishment and proliferation of health planning agencies. By the early 1960s the most common were still voluntary in nature. At that time these organizations, commonly known as areawide health planning agencies, were generally either traditional hospital membership organizations or community-centered agencies. The release of substantial amounts of federal funds intended to help further organize health care planning in many cities led to closer government scrutiny and control. Guidelines were developed by a joint committee of the American Hospital Association and the United States Public Health Service in 1961.[14] The following principles were suggested. Key public or private agencies were expected to take the initiative in establishing planning units where they did not presently exist. Governing bodies of agencies should be comprised of community leaders, not to include substantial numbers of full-time health workers. It was recommended that these agencies be established on a permanent basis. The agencies were expected to have official Hill-Burton sanctions for operating. Geographic regions normally centered about one or more cities and incorporating SMSA's were delimited. Areawide health planning agencies were asked to develop profiles of all health care facilities within their specified geographic regions. They were also expected to collect information about the communities they served, including demographic, socioeconomic, and population at risk indicators. They were also

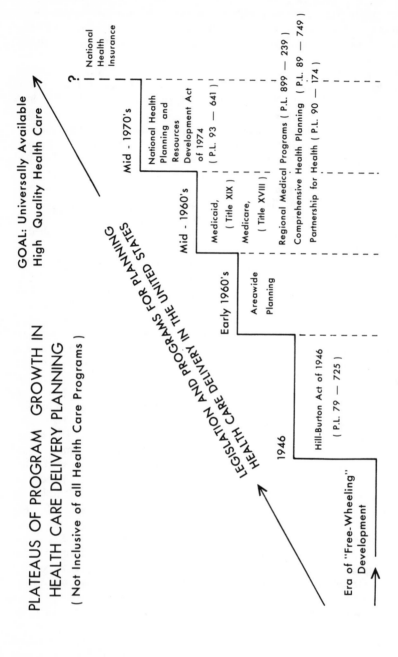

Fig. 96. Various plateaus of program growth in health care planning from 1946 to 1978 in the United States. Not all major health care programs are included.

required to develop profiles of health care facilities that would include information about obsolescence, distributions of services developed by patient origin studies, educational programs, and distributions of other health-related resources.

These guidelines were followed by many agencies already in existence and new ones that were created. Many problems developed. Because of the voluntary nature of areawide health planning agencies at that time there was often a lack of cooperation from state Hill–Burton agencies. On many occasions there was general reluctance on the part of many hospitals to supply information to the planning agencies. In many locations areawide planning agencies could not obtain the needed cooperation from medical and hospital associations. There was an overall lack of representation on the governing boards of the agencies from the general community. In spite of these shortcomings, since dispersement of public monies required the development of plans, many comprehensive plans of a sophisticated nature resulted. These plans differed from one planning agency to another and there was a lack of any standardized national format.

Included within the massive barrage of social legislation in the mid-1960s were many programs geared toward improving health status and health planning. In retrospect, the two with the greatest impact on health status, and eventually health planning programs, were Medicaid and Medicare (Titles XVIII and XIX of the Social Security Act). Joint federal–state efforts, Medicaid programs are intended to provide medical care to public assistance recipients and others who do not qualify for public aid but are unable to pay for medical care. Programs are administered by state agencies and the national government provides varying proportions of the costs. Medicaid coverage includes a wide variety of health care costs, the most important of which are inpatient and outpatient hospital service and physician care. Medicare provides similar coverage for the elderly. These two programs have contributed much since their inception to the health care needs of the indigent and elderly, and they have also contributed substantially to our need for improved health care planning programs.

Also included in the mid-1960s legislation were the Regional Medical Programs, created by Public Law 89-239 in 1965, and a new basis for reorganization in health planning in the form of the Comprehensive Health Planning Act of 1966 (Public Law 89-749). Destined to be shortlived, the Regional Medical Programs were categorical in nature, with an overall goal of developing programs to combat heart disease, cancer, and stroke.[15] One of the many problems confronting Regional Medical Programs nationally was a lack of overall cooperation and organization. In a *laissez faire* fashion it was left to local areas to develop Regional Medical Programs and subsequently carve out their own territories (see Figure 97). Geographic boundaries of Regional Medical Programs were never clearly defined on a national basis. In some instances they included one or more states, and in others consisted of one complete state and parts of one or more others. Some Regional Medical Programs claimed several states and their planning areas overlapped with other regional medical programs. Some were parts of states and still others were exclusively metropolitan.

Following the requirements of Public Law 89-749, Comprehensive Health Planning Agencies under various titles were developed in metropolitan locations

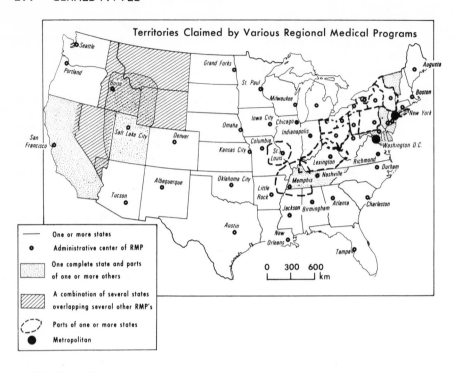

Fig. 97. Different territories claimed by Regional Medical Programs in the United States prior to the termination of the program nationally.

in the United States. In some places previously established voluntary areawide health planning agencies assumed the role of Comprehensive Health Planning Agencies. Upon occasion, some health planning agencies carried on the functions of Regional Medical Programs as well as those separately established by the Comprehensive Health Planning Act. One of the initial intents of establishing Comprehensive Health Planning Agencies was to create authorities vested to review applications for new health care delivery developments. Strong competition arose between Regional Medical Programs and Comprehensive Health Planning Agencies. In essence, a contradiction existed because there was duplication in the existence of health planning agencies. Regional Medical Programs were terminated in the mid-1970s. The termination of Regional Medical Programs offered Comprehensive Health Planning Agencies the opportunity to become the "official" health planning bodies in their designated areas.

In 1974 the National Health Planning and Resources Development Act (Public Law 93-641) was passed. For many practitioners in health care facilities planning, this legislation was the long-awaited panacea to their problems. In many respects this act was an extension, refinement, and clarification of the Comprehensive Health Planning Act of 1966. Even before the 1974 legislation, such terms as "provider" and "consumer" had become meaningful concepts to health planners. Because in many instances so many of the members of the boards of earlier areawide health planning agencies were somehow associated with the provision of health care, this dichotomized relationship (provider vs. consumer) was developed to eliminate the problem of vested self-interests in planning for health care facilities. Over the past decade many terms, abbreviations, and acronyms have developed as an outgrowth of health planning legislation program development and practice. Appendix A has been included in the last part of this book as a glossary of terms now being used by health planning agencies. Reference to the glossary assists in comprehending the terms used currently in health planning practice and the interrelationships of various levels of health planning.[16]

The 1974 legislation had two major portions. The first part was intended to update existing health planning programs. The second was intended to revise existing programs for the construction and modernization of health-care facilities and replaced the then outdated Hill–Burton program. In addition, the legislation called for funds to be dispersed to local health-planning agencies for the implementation of their plans. The legislation required that the Secretary of the Department of Health, Education, and Welfare issue guidelines concerning national health planning policy.[17] At this time many guidelines have been issued. The legislation established much more than viable local planning agencies with review authority. It called for cooperation among the Secretary of DHEW, state health planning agencies and local agencies. Statewide health coordinating councils were also established. In effect, the program called for a network of Health Systems Agencies (HSA's) responsible for health planning and development throughout the country. Within each state, Governors subsequently designated health service areas for purposes of planning. The requirements included that designated areas be reasonably appropriate for effective planning, and were based on such factors as population and availability of resources to provide necessary health services. With some exceptions, Health Systems Agencies were expected to have a population of not less than 500,000 nor more than 3,000,000, and whenever possible boundaries would be coordinated with other regional planning areas. The entire country was eventually exhausted geographically (see Figure 98) with Health Systems Agencies representing either expanded or contracted boundaries of former Comprehensive Health Planning Agencies.[18] In structuring these service areas it was intended that SMSA boundaries not be violated; however, when SMSA's straddled state boundaries, exceptions were made. HSA's were tasked to gather and analyze information suitable for planning purposes within their boundaries. They were mandated to establish Health Systems Plans (HSP) and annual implementation plans (AIP). The legislation specified that they were to coordinate activities with Professional Standards Review Organizations (PSRO's) and other appropriate planning and regulatory entities. They were empowered to review and approve or disapprove applications for federal funds for health programs within their designated areas, and further tasked to assist states in the performance of capital expenditures

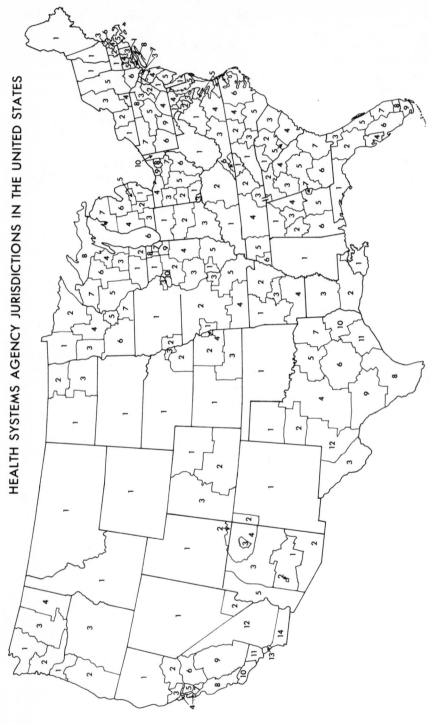

Fig. 98. Jurisdictions of Health Systems Agencies in the United States in 1978.

reviews. These and other functions have now come to fruition as various Health Systems Agencies throughout the United States reach the status of being "designated" as official health planning bodies.

At the state level designated health planning agencies were designated to be advised by a Statewide Health Coordinating Council (SHCC). Requirements for these councils included that at least 60% of their membership be appointed by the Governor of the state's Health Systems Agencies and have a consumer majority. These councils were mandated to annually review and coordinate Health Systems Plans (HSP's) and Annual Implementation Plans (AIP's) of the state's Health Systems Agencies and make comments to the Secretary of Health, Education, and Welfare. In addition, the councils are expected to prepare state plans made up of the Health Systems Plans of the various local agencies taking into account a preliminary plan developed by the state agencies. Other functions expected are: a review of budgets and applications for financial assistance from local agencies; advising the state agency on the performance of its functions; and review and approval or disapproval of state health plans and applications for formula grants to the state.

One part of the 1974 legislation provided that the Secretary of DHEW may make grants for purposes of demonstrating the effectiveness of rate regulation to a number of states choosing to accomplish regulation. Other general provisions included procedures and criteria for the use of local and state agencies in performing reviews required by the act. The legislation also provided that the Secretary of DHEW offer technical assistance to local and state agencies and establish a national health planning information center. A provision was included to designate one university in each of the DHEW regions as a resource center for health planning. It was further required that the Secretary of DHEW review and act upon annual budgets of local and state agencies and develop performance standards for the agencies. A plethora of additional stipulations were included in the act, some of the most meaningful pertained to authority of review in local areas pertaining to modernization of medical facilities, construction of new outpatient and inpatient facilities and conversions of existing medical facilities. The act went so far as to authorize local health planning agencies to review applications by hospitals for certain kinds of costly equipment. Actual review procedures are discussed later in this chapter.

Guidelines recently issued pertaining to the establishment of information bases by local agencies are particularly important because they expect geographical data inputs: including population at risk indicators, health status indicators, and health services, and resources indicators. The role of medical geographers in the provision of health planning information is by no means a recent phenomenon. As each plateau of program growth in health care delivery planning evolved over the past several decades, geographers have become increasingly involved at various levels in health planning practice. Initial and subsequent involvements of geographers are an outgrowth of the application of general principles of location theory.

Hierarchies of Facilities and Resources?

Shannon and Dever offer an optimal model for spatial and functional arrangement in planning for the delivery of health care.[19] The general model, the context of central place theory, suggests that initial providers of health care (physicians) be locationally spaced to serve maximum numbers of people within reasonable distances. This would also hold true for group practices and clinics. Since smaller hospitals logically have smaller areas of service, and these service areas increase with hospital size, it is optimally possible to place an entire hierarchy of facilities within a space-maximizing spatial mosaic. Because few populations are distributed evenly over uniform planes, necessary modifications to such arrangements are expected. The Swedes have probably most closely approximated this kind of spatial-functional planning. It is within the context of central place theory and related concepts of locational analysis that some of the earliest contributions in health care geography can be found. Examples include Godlund's work pertaining to hospital use and transportation facilities in Sweden and that of Garrison, et al. addressing highway development and geographic change.[20]

Aspects of transportation, distance, and hospital size play an important role in the development of these dynamic spatial allocation models. In a 1969 contribution Shannon et al. suggested the use of a modified gravity model in explaining the relationship between the distance from place of residence and hospital location utilized by patients.[21] Attempts have been made to apply this model and other variants, but with large samples of hosptials and frequent overlap in service areas due to hospital clusters, actual allocations of patients to hospitals cannot account for individual choice behavior in many circumstances. It is possible to incorporate some aspects of behavior with travel time and distance, and this was accomplished by Earickson in 1970.[22] Earickson came to the conclusions that solutions of the transportation problem in formal terms, game theory, and gravity constraints, cannot offer comprehensive explanations of hospital service areas. As a result, he developed a simulation model to account for additional variables including intervening opportunities and racial and religious behavior. Following this logic of allocation model development, hospital size has been identified as a key variable in understanding service areas. Morrill and Earickson found that a gravity or power model similar to that suggested by Shannon was more appropriate for explaining the service area of medium to small general hospitals, but larger hospitals with more specialities demonstrated service areas that tended to fit a generalized negative exponential function.[23]

The gravity and exponential models have become the two most competitive for such dynamic analyses. Some disagreement has developed pertaining to which approach is more appropriate. Still, there are obvious similarities between the two, and this occurs because of the use of the distance component. In some descriptions of hospital service areas, distance decay mechanisms, the effects of hospital size, intervening opportunities and other determinants of hospital use can be incorporated through market penetration models.[24] The use of optimum time-distance allocation models is especially important to methodologies intended to establish locations for emergency medical services.[25] Within this context, the allocation models become more than descriptive tools. If properly utilized in the planning process, lives as well as capital can be saved. More coordination in health care planning to include these concepts is required.

Unfortunately in most parts of the United States the idealized functional-spatial optimal relationship among various levels of the health care delivery system does not exist. It is possible to identify some spatial aspects of the hierarchical nature of these facilities, particularly among hospitals. As a general rule, the size of the area served by a hospital increases with hospital size. This relationship for most of the hospitals in the Chicago metropolitan area is shown within Figure 99. The slope of the relationship is nearly a perfect straight line. The larger hospitals with the higher average daily census are major research and regional hospitals. The cluster of smaller ones tends to be medium-sized city hospitals and smaller hospitals. As part of the five-year Chicago Regional Hospital Study efforts, Morrill and Earickson identified a hierarchy of hospitals within the

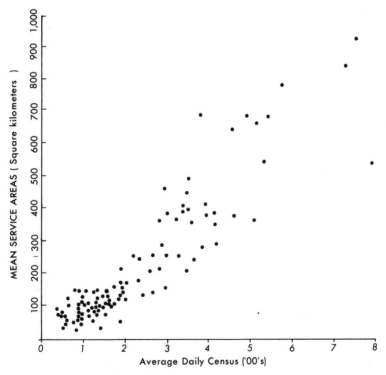

Fig. 99. The extent of hospital service areas in relation to average daily census. This graph shows the general hierarchical nature of systems of hospitals.

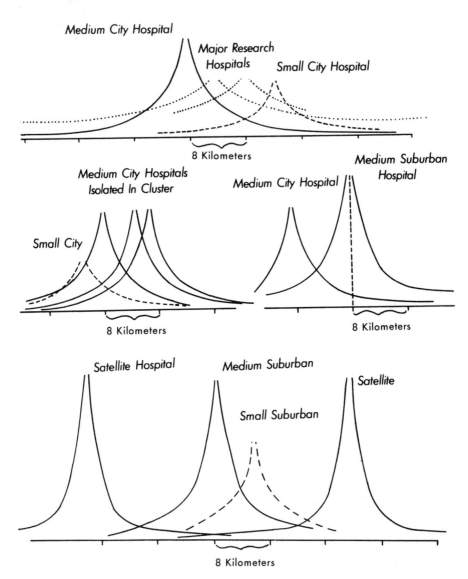

Fig. 100. Size and shape of demand cones for different kinds of hospitals in the Chicago area.

Chicago area.[26] Major research hospitals, all affiliated with medical schools, demonstrated a wide spatial range of services corresponding with the large numbers of facilities available. Regional hospitals with some linkages to medical schools and large staffs also demonstrated very large service areas. The service area relationships among these and other kinds of hospitals are depicted by the "demand cones" shown within Figure 100. Those considered community hospitals were further subdivided into three groups: large community nonspecialized hospitals; community hospitals with some specialization; and smaller community hospitals. The service areas within this group displayed some variance depending upon hospital location. Satellite hospitals, for example, tended to have steeper slopes than most other kinds. Some of the suburban community hospitals had slopes almost as steep as those of inner-city hospitals, in the same general hierarchical class. Clusters of hospitals of this type in the inner city showed combined service areas. Smaller suburban and inner-city hospitals, having more difficulty attracting staff and patients, showed correspondingly smaller service areas. Exceptions to the above patterns could be found in communities where single hospitals have virtual monopolies.

Two key factors in understanding the use of hospitals as major health care delivery resources consist of location of the facilities and size. Aside from the sophisticated hierarchical formulations used in the Chicago Regional Hospital Study, hospitals are normally categorized in size ranges depending upon the number of available hospital beds. In a patient origin study accomplished in 1973 in part of northeastern Ohio, it was possible to develop a regional composite of hospital service areas as information to be used in the planning process.[27] The study area shown within Figure 101 serves as an example of the arrangement of hospital service areas in a six-county region. The counties range in size from Stark, the largest with 380,000 people (1975 estimate) to Holmes with 25,000 people (1975). Stark County is part of the Canton SMSA and a major manufacturing and retail center. Note the significant overlap in the service areas of four hospitals within the most urbanized Stark County portion of the study area. Another method of demonstrating this overlap is the southwest to northeast cross-section of the distance decay functions representing the service areas of the hospitals in the county. Aultman and Timken are the two largest hospitals with approximately 600 and 500 beds, respectively. Massillon and Doctors' Hospital are in the medium range with approximately 200 and 250 beds. Alliance Hospital, located in an industrial satellite community in the extreme northeastern part of the county, normally functions with about 165 beds. Due to its location, somewhat removed from the urban core of the county, Alliance Hospital has a much more extensive service area than those located in Canton.

Other forms of service area overlap also were identified in that part of Ohio. For example, Figure 102 contains distance-decay profiles of overlapping services areas in Wayne and Richland Counties. The hospitals in Wayne County include Wooster (159 beds), Dunlap (55 beds), and Wayne Hospital (42 beds). The latter two hospitals are considered by most definitions to be small, while Wooster Hosptial is in the medium range. However, the profiles for Wooster and Dunlap Hospitals are nearly identical in terms of catchment. Wayne Hospital

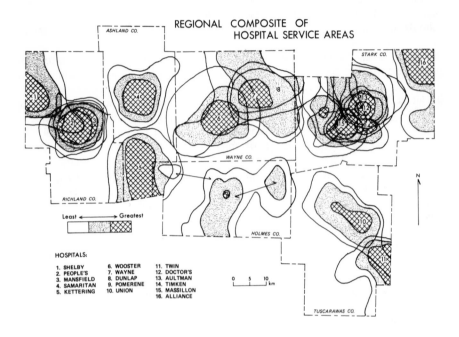

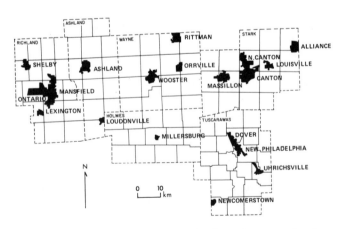

Fig. 101. A regional composite of hospital service areas in six counties in part of Northeastern Ohio.

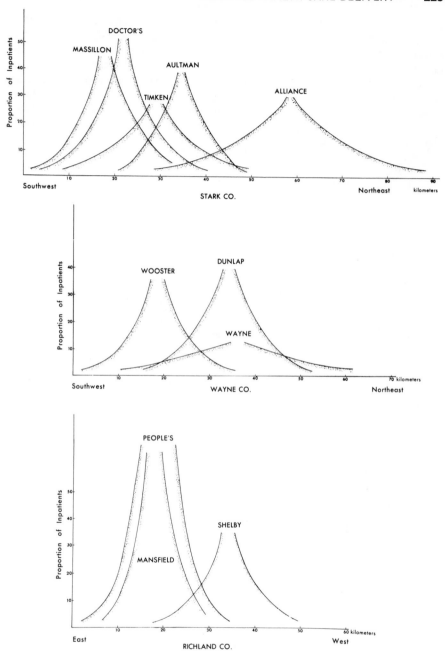

Fig. 102. Demand cones showing various degrees of overlap in heavily urban and moderately settled counties.

demonstrated a very shallow distance-decay relationship, and its service area is almost entirely subsumed by the other two hospitals. An analogous situation is indicated when distance-decay relationships for the three hospitals in Richland County are compared (see Figure 102). The service area of Mansfield Hospital is completely incorporated within that of People's Hospital, while the Shelby Hospital service area shows some overlap but also major catchment to the west.

Ashland and Tuscarawas Counties contain hospitals with locational attributes closer to what might be considered more optimal for purposes of health planning. Figure 103 indicates that there is little overlap in Ashland County for the service areas of Kettering and Samaritan hospitals. Both Kettering and Samaritan hospitals are considered small in terms of numbers of beds. Somewhat more overlap is apparent when viewing the distance-decay relationship for Twin

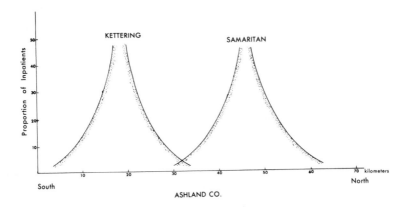

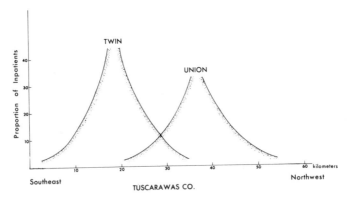

Fig. 103. Overlap of demand cones in moderate to sparsely settled areas.

and Union Hospitals in Tuscarawas County. These hospitals are considered medium to small.

Some of this information was used by the Health Planning and Development Council of Wooster, Ohio (the Health Systems Agency of that region) in determining future needs for the region. As with many agencies, a variant of the older Hill-Burton formula was utilized:

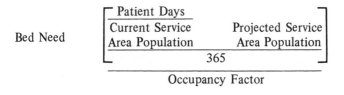

Where Occupancy Factors are,

1) Medical–Surgical Units > 250 Beds = 90%,
2) Medical–Surgical Units < 250 Beds = 85%,
3) Obstretical Units   < 250 Beds = 75%, and
4) Pediatric Units   = 75%.

This method was used to provide an estimate of bed need for a time period extending into 1985. Needs were then compared to actual occupancy statistics. The information will prove to be useful as hospitals apply for approval of various projects.

The clustering of hospital service areas within more highly urbanized locations requires more detailed spatial analysis than that offered from the above example. In a 1975 study, the effects of overlapping hospital service areas were analyzed for part of the Akron, Ohio SMSA.[28] In this example, a market penetration model was calibrated by determining the relationship between numbers of patients utilizing three hospitals in the four to six hundred bed range. All are located within a few kilometers of one another (see Figure 104). Examination of the individual service areas of the three individual hospitals indicates definite forms of distance and directional bias. For example, St. Thomas Hospital with about 400 beds available at that time and the smallest of the three had a service area extending northward from the central city of Akron. Part of this configuration was due to transportation barriers to the south as well as methods of physician referral from the north. The service area for Akron General Medical Center, a regional hospital with approximately 550 beds, also demonstrated an assymetrical shape. The parts of the study area with the largest proportion of inpatients formed in a corridor extending northwest of the hospital into suburban locations. Akron City Hospital, by far the largest with 635 beds and the most specialities, had the largest service area of the three. That service area included two cores, one encompassing most of the city of Akron and extending to the southeast and the other in northwestern Akron. In addition, Akron City Hospital

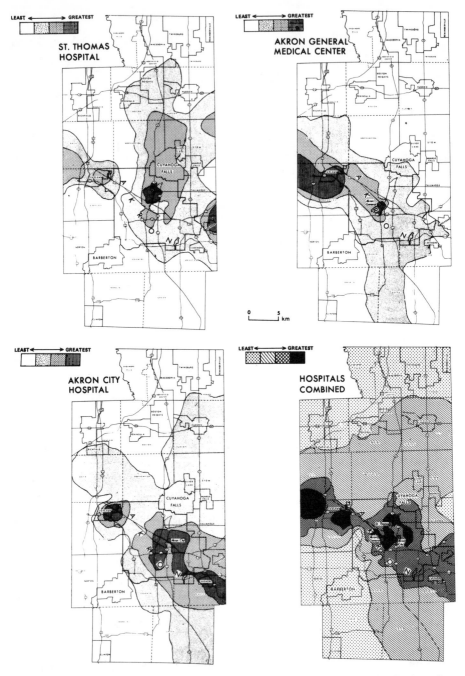

Fig. 104. Hospital Market Penetration Levels. This illustration shows three hospital service areas separately and in combination.

also serves most of the eastern suburbs within the county. It proved useful in this comparison to recalibrate the market penetration model and construct a service area showing the three hospitals combined. The results indicated two areas of heaviest market penetration in and around the central city (also where the population is most dense) and two areas of concentration to the northwest. The indentation in the southwest is due to the presence of a hospital in Barberton, thus reflecting that intervening opportunity.

In general, it is possible to understand more about clustered urban hospitals by examination of service areas in the aggregate than from investigation of each service area separately. This also proves to be true in statistical terms. Distance-decay relationships for each of the three hospitals individually and the combined service area best fit the exponential model. Expected regularities were discovered. St. Thomas, the smallest hospital with a heavily northern suburban fetch, demonstrated the weakest fit ($R = -.36$). Since the slope was less steep than the others, the directional bias of the service area could be expressed in comparative measurable terms. The exponential function for Akron General Medical Center ($R = -.64$) was substantially better than St. Thomas and this would be expected considering hospital size. Among the three hospitals the best fit was with Akron City, the largest ($R = -.71$). Not unexpectedly, an even better fit was obtained when the market penetration of the combined hospitals was formulated ($R = -.72$). These relationships are shown within Figure 105.

Subsequent investigations indicated that the hospital service areas were also influenced to some extent by physician referral habits, particularly in areas of strong overlap. Since detailed diagnostic referral data were not available, and this is often the case in such analyses, a canonical factor analysis similar to the method indicated within Chapter 6 was used to compare reported mortality data with a variety of health status indicators. Leading causes of death were most strongly associated statistically with indicators of generally lower socioeconomic status and income. By subdividing the county study area into six broad geographic-socioeconomic groups, it was possible to compare hospital use with urban ecological units (the methodology was similar to those discussed within Chapter 6). Average mortality rates for heart disease, cancer, and stroke within each ecological group generally followed trends reported over the years by many health researchers. The ecological group with the least resources appeared to be most affected by major leading causes of death, and the group with the most resources was least affected. In fact, when comparing all six groups, a systematic scale consisting of high mortality/least resources to low mortality/most resources was identified among the six groups. When hospital use for the groups was also analyzed the results were not quite the same. The lowest resource, low income, urban ecological group manifested substantially more proportionate hospital use than the group with the most resources. Part of this phenomenon is definitely due to the availability and use of Medicaid and Medicare programs. The ecological group that deviated most from what otherwise might have been a regularity inversely related to mortality patterns and hospital use was second to lowest on the resource scale. Parts of the city comprising this urban ecological group accounted for relatively lower rates of hospital use than expected. While

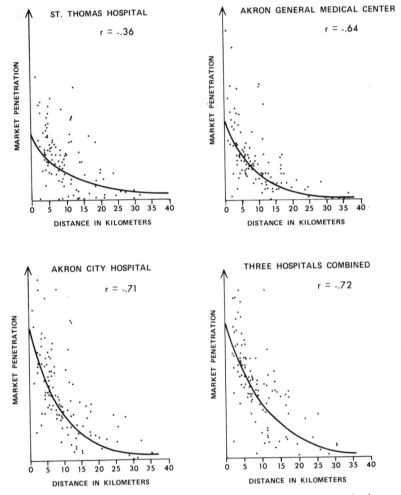

Fig. 105. Distance-decay relationships for the three hospitals shown in Figure 104 and a combined fit.

the effects of sociomedical legislation could be seen operating with lowest income groups along with other forms of health care payment coverage playing a role as necessary with subsequently higher resource groups, there appeared to be a "crack" in the delivery system. When this happens it can be described as a condition wherein many persons who are marginally poor or of modest means but cannot qualify for federal programs frequently cannot muster the financial resources sufficient to pay for hospital treatment. This results in what some might term an underdemand. The condition also raises a number of questions pertaining to use of physicians and other forms of health care seeking behavior.

In 1976 Shannon and Spurlock offered a methodology for examining the behavior of various societal groups within the context of what they termed "urban ecological containers and environmental risk cells" in the use of medical services.[29] Based on a survey in the Washington, D.C. area, their information base was more detailed than the data available for the Akron study mentioned above. They suggested that it is more appropriate in such comparisons to define environmental risk cells than to attempt to isolate natural disease foci. They proposed the identification of high environmental risk cells consisting of parts of cities exposed to health hazards more than the average. Their methodology offers ways to construct definitions of ranges of such proportionately different risk cells. Utilizing the standard elipse methodology developed by Lefever,[30] they compared hospital use among various socioeconomic groups with other definitions of behavioral space. Their results indicated forms of spatial mismatch when medical care areas were compared to the other forms of activity space. Part of the imbalance was due to the uneven distribution of medical care opportunities. Yet another factor was explained as different uses of geographic space by various urban ecological groups. Application of this methodology leads to meaningful results when survey data are available.

In a more recent contribution Shannon explored the conceptual organization of space, time, and illness behavior and offered a framework for more comprehensive investigation in medical geography.[31] Shannon explained how individuals often, but not always, on the basis of group behavior, develop operational domains within settlements. He suggests the integration of Fabrega's model of illness behavior into a proposed geographic methodology including:[32] illness recognition and labeling; illness disvalues; treatment plans; assessment of treatment plans; evaluation of potential treatment benefits; treatment costs; potential net benefits; selection of treatment plan; and a possible recycling of these items in some systematic fashion. In essence, the illness behavioral model depends upon perceived severity of symptoms, family responses, possible medical-psychological systems, accompanying behavioral changes and treatment actions. When Fabrega's system of behavior is interwoven with known theoretical aspects of perception of geographic space, an important framework for analysis can be developed. Within the context of this proposed model, Shannon considers mortality data a poor index of health status because of possible differences in the availability or quality of treatment. He strongly recommends, instead, the sophisticated use of survey techniques and medical sampling. This approach to understanding human use of medical services can be applied by medical geographers. In addition, the survey method has become a major tool for systematic collection of health-related data, and several worthwhile methodologies have recently been put forth by the National Center for Health Services Research.[33]

Spatial studies of the use of health care resources often produce results indicating various forms of maldistribution or imbalance, and almost regardless of method of data acquisition this appers to be particularly true in analyses of physician distributions. DeVise has contended that once M.D.'s complete their medical education they are often attracted to parts of the United States with higher income potential or more pleasant climate.[34] In a more detailed comparison of physician location behavior, Shannon and Dever have offered several overlapping explanations.[35] Important factors considered in such behavior include population, income, the availability of medical facilities, and the presence of medical education institutions. Prime considerations also include the availability of medical research facilities, a demand on the part of physicians for ancillary health care personnel and facilities, and perceived opportunities to eventually interact in medical education. In spite of these possible macroscale determinants other forces can be seen operating within metropolitan areas. In an analysis of the changing distribution of private practice physician office locations in the Chicago area from 1950 to 1970, Dewey identified several factors contributing to change.[36] Dewey discovered that for over a period of two decades the distribution of physicians' offices had gradually shifted away from the commerical core of Chicago and parts of the inner city into suburbs. The shift in office locations was also away from racially changing neighborhoods. Locations within proximity to newly planned suburban retail shopping centers appeared attractive to many physicians. Other factors included the type of medical specialization of the physician and the size and variety of services provided by adjacent hospitals. In an earlier contribution, Lubin et al. suggested that factors requiring examination in such comparisons include the number of hospitals a physician might use in relation to the distribution of his patients, types of available hospital services, actual distances physicians would have to travel to and from hospitals, and travel time within major metropolitan areas.[37] The latter aspect does vary considerably. While Dewey's study showed physician office locations "following" populations to selected suburban locations, Rosenthal contends that such movement reflects the effects of population density and change.[38] Utilizing two counties in Florida, a state with a higher than average ratio of physicians to population, Rosenthal found that the physician population in Broward and Palm Beach Counties was growing faster than the general population rate of increase. There were proportionately more specialists than general practitioners. Locations of physicians' offices generally followed population change and growth. In general, part of this kind of location behavior is a natural response for proprietary retail establishments.

The problem of unbalanced distributions of physicians in relation to the population at the national as well as the local levels is certainly the result of a physician shortage in the United States. Nothing short of substantially increasing the number of medical education facilities throughout the country will solve the problem. While necessary, such a solution is long-term in nature. More immediate responses have resulted in modified forms of increasing physician availability. Some are programmatic in origin and others follow the American *laissez faire* approach to health care delivery.

One such concept is the Health Maintenance Organization proposed during the Republican administration of the early 1970s. While the term HMO appeared to be unique, the actual concept was an outgrowth of a trend toward specialized prepaid group practice operations.[39] Simply defined, health care delivered is "prepaid." Members of these organizations prepay specified fees at regular intervals regardless of the amount of health care treatment utilized. The concept dates to the turn of this century in its origins when members of organized labor groups, including the Ladies Garment Workers Union of New York, bargained for fringe benefits. Similar programs subsequently were successful in locations far removed from urban and more populated settlements where health care services were more readily available.[40] In areas with mining and logging activities, prepaid group practices were initiated. At construction sites in the West the Kaiser Corporation developed prepaid programs. After World War II a Kaiser Foundation Health Plan began to serve individuals not directly employed by Kaiser Industries. The concept diffused to other West Coast locations, and many similar groups were formed in California. Ideally, such a method of health care delivery can benefit the physician and the patient. It is possible for physicians in most forms of group practice to be less overworked because of the sharing of responsibilities and peer consultation. The patient is more or less guaranteed quicker access to a physician. While an attempt was made to offer the HMO as a national program, partially as an alternative to national health insurance, it was not successful for many reasons. After the program was put forth in the form of a proposed national policy, virtually no geographic factors were considered in the planning process. Applications for HMO status were purely on a voluntary basis. As would be expected, substantial numbers of group practices in the western United States applied for HMO status. Some already successful urban prepaid group practices qualified as Health Maintenance Organizations. The most successful of the latter was the Health Insurance Plan (HIP) of Greater New York. The HIP group opened its doors in 1947 and by the late 1960s had incorporated Medicaid and Medicare payments into its program. In addition to lack of spatial considerations in planning, the entire program did not consider enough aspects of universal medical care. Prepaid group practice patients, for example, are often preselected and annual physicals are required. The focus on preventive health care is admirable, but restrictions automatically exclude people who already have serious health problems and are in need of immediate treatment.

The basic concept of physician group practice is viable in health care delivery. With proper planning it can also be spatially efficient. There is a movement within the United States in the health care industry to establish more family group practice centers often administratively affiliated with hospitals. Still, there are insufficient manpower resources to develop a comprehensive national network of such centers.

As physician location and travel behavior have changed historically, the entire concept of house calls has become a virtual relic. We now refer to ambulatory care as consisting of health services provided on an outpatient basis. This term usually implies that patients travel to locations to receive services and depart the same day. Forms of ambulatory care consist of the types of delivery mentioned above: proprietary, solo, and group practices. Ambulatory care now also takes the form of outpatient departments based either within hospitals or as satellite operations.[41] Spatial aspects of patient behavior closely approximate inpatient hospital use. Traditionally, outpatient hospital departments served the poor, usually in the form of emergency rooms, clinics and certain supporting services. With the physician shortage and the inauguration of health care programs nationally for the medically indigent, the distinction between clinical services and emergency room services became increasingly difficult to make for a period of time. Given the current trend toward the formation of group practices, aspects of changes in population structure, including a higher median age and lower fertility rates, along with programmatic developments leading toward more adequate methods of payment, the form and function of many hospitals are changing. Lower birth rates and more stringent regulatory measures have led to declines in hospital maternity and obstetrical departments. Since hospitals are a large capital investment and not footloose in terms of location choice, they generally do not move. Architectural and construction alterations make use of available space in many instances.

While hospitals are also regulated in terms of the addition of new beds, forms of new construction (sometimes physical additions) quite often consist of outpatient departments separated from emergency rooms. Such a separation allows more use of emergency rooms for their intended purpose. These forms of change also alleviate the problem of attempting to limit emergency room use and tend to project the role of the hospital as a community health center offering ambulatory care.[42] This expanded role of the hospital fills in some spatial gaps in the ambulatory care level of the health care delivery hierarchy. However, since the trend is at this time not progammatical in a policy sense, outpatient hospital departments are spatially constrained to predetermine locations. An optimal central place theoretic network of health care provision, if this is indeed an ideal form, does not appear to be either possible or practical with this form of health care delivery.

Many specialized forms of ambulatory care have been available within hospitals for some time. Geographic patterns of patient use of these specialized services have traditionally been determined by physician referral patterns, sometimes regardless of distance. Through utilization of many of the geographic principles discussed within this chapter, it is possible to develop health care delivery planning models for these services. One such model which proved to be spatially efficient but economically impractical was a disease categorical allocation procedure developed for cancer radiation therapy treatment in the Chicago metropolitan area.[43] The effort was part of the Regional Medical Program effort and the aim was to spatially allocate forecasted patients requiring teletherapy treatments to optimal locations. The optimizing procedure also included general economic constraints. In general, the process consisted of forecasting need for teletherapy treatment ahead one decade. An allocation model was then used to assign patients to existing teletherapy units. The allocation procedure incorporated distance constraints and some limited behavioral aspects in health care seeking. As the existing units reached reasonable capacities through allocations of numbers of new and existing patients, the residual forecasted patients were considered a geographic expression of unmet need. Hospitals both with and without existing teletherapy installations were examined within the context of an overall cost curve (see Figure 106). It was discovered that the absence or presence of a teletherapy unit made no difference with respect to a hospital's position along the overall cost curve. Hospitals without installations and no extreme deviation from average costs were considered as potential locations for the installation of new teletherapy units. The overall cost-curve position of these hospitals is shown within Figure 107. Geographic concentrations of projected unmet need were examined in conjunction with transportation access, and those

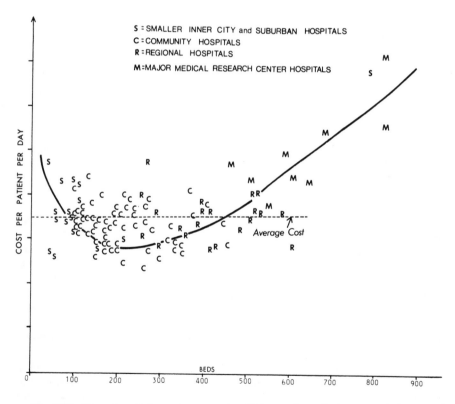

Fig. 106. The hospital cost curve in Chicago in relation to 4 kinds of institutions.

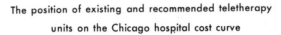

The position of existing and recommended teletherapy
units on the Chicago hospital cost curve

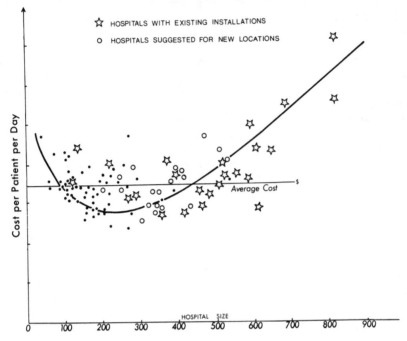

Fig. 107. Use of the cost curve as one ingredient in planning for the location of new teletherapy installations.

locations shown within Figure 108 were recommended as optimal new locations for teletherapy installations.

In actual practice, the locational plan was not fully put into effect. The major reasons were economics and policy. For example, the actual new patient cost effective threshold used at that time was about half the minimum 500 new patients a year subsequently incorporated into health planning legislation. Since capital expenditures for this kind of cancer treatment equipment are substantial, the inclusion of new installations and accompanying programs now falls under the review authority of Health Systems Agencies. A general method of assessing community needs for radiation therapy treatment consists of inventorying all facilities within a Health Systems Area and comparing the number of units in ratio form to the total population. Geographical location frequently does not become a consideration, especially when communities have more treatment installations than the prescribed monotonic ratio. In some instances teletherapy units have been closed down for this reason. One rationale for using this

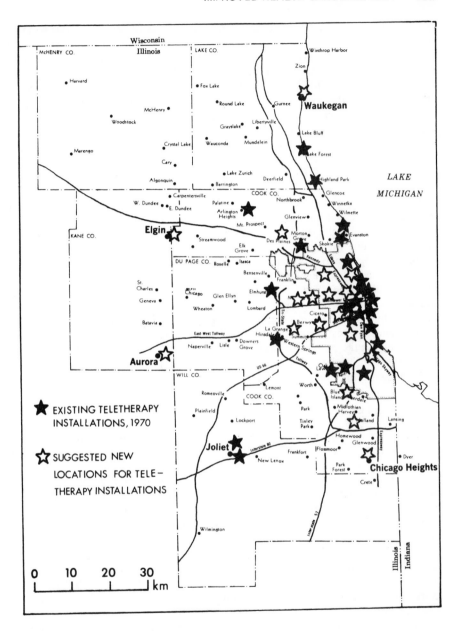

Fig. 108. Existing and suggested locations for teletherapy installations in the Chicago metropolitan area for the 1970s.

approach is economic. The logic followed is fairly straightforward. If this form of perceived duplication exists for many forms of medical equipment, the entire population of an area eventually pays for the added costs. The reader is reminded that aspects of duplication of services and societal diseconomics predate the Hill–Burton Act of 1946. Cost and policy have since become interwoven into the logic of health care delivery planning. Paradoxically, after three decades of health care delivery planning program development, cost has become more important than ever.

THE REALITIES OF COST AND POLICY

With perhaps the exceptions of planning for optimal emergency medical services delivery and the development of spatial-functional health care delivery hierarchies in emerging nations, the role of the medical geographer in health care delivery planning must be expanded to incorporate economic and policy changes. A theoretically practical optimal allocation solution may often not be practical because of economic realities. While independent or semiindependent research in an academic vacuum can easily lead to the identification of geographic inequalities, findings cannot be translated into action easily if they depart substantially from existing planning policy. Scientific research has never directed public policy in health care planning to a major degree. Also, the economic crisis the United States currently faces in health care has influenced planning policy and subsequently determined research directions. The extent of the economic problem cannot be underestimated.

An Economic Crisis

Health care costs are largely determined by the amount of various services purchased and the price of these services. Quantities of health services delivered have changed with changes in characteristics of the U.S. population. Utilization patterns have also become altered among various population groups because of program developments. Accelerated recent growth in overall national health expenditures has been primarily attributed to increases in prices.[44] Compiled and published annually by the Social Security Administration, measures of national health expenditures include costs incurred in the delivery of health care, administration of health care programs, construction of health-related facilities and biomedical and other health-related research. In 1976 the total amount spent for such programs in the United States was almost 140 billion dollars, or an average of about $640 dollars per person. This represented 8.6% of the nation's GNP.[45] For purposes of comparison of the changing proportion of the GNP devoted to health spending from 1950 to 1975 refer to Figure 109. The percent of the GNP expended on health care will soon double the amount of 1950. The annual rate of growth in national health expenditures has now exceeded the growth in expenditures for most other goods and services. There has been a steady upward trend since 1950, but increases in the late 1970s approach exponential proportions.

NATIONAL HEALTH EXPENDITURES 1950 — 1975

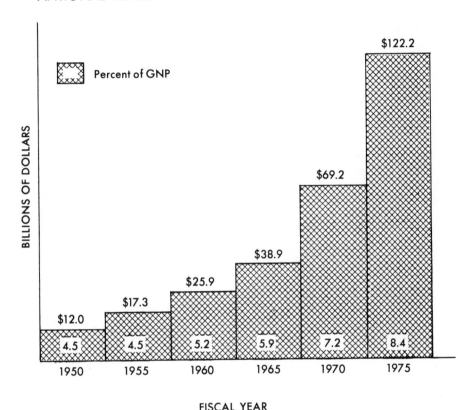

FISCAL YEAR

Source: Social Security Administration

Fig. 109. Growing health care expenditures in the United States from 1950 to 1975.

Part of the cost problem can be attributed to inflation, but part is also because of the changing pattern of health care financing. In 1950 the government paid 20% of the cost for personal health care expenditures. By 1975 that proportion had doubled (see Figure 110). In contrast, 68% of all personal health care payments in the United States in 1950 were by direct payment. In 1975 direct payment accounted for 34%, or exactly half that amount. These are the two most notable trends: government expenditures have proportionately doubled and direct payment has exactly halved. Charity payments have always played a small role, but a noticeable change has taken place from 3% of all payments in

PERSONAL HEALTH CARE EXPENDITURES 1950 — 1975

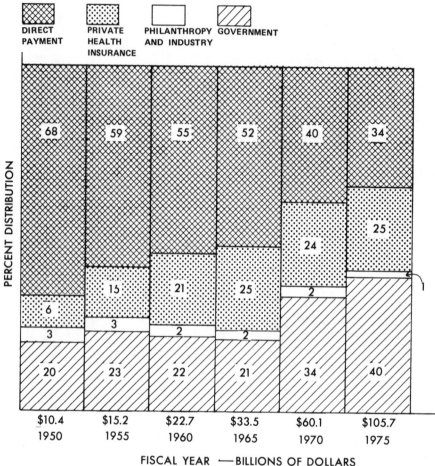

Fig. 110. The changing composition of method of payment in the United States from 1950 to 1975.

1950 to approximately 1% in 1975. By 1960 private health insurance had accounted for approximately one-fifth of all payments and this has risen somewhat to about a quarter by the mid-1970s. Much of the increased government expenditures are due to public payment programs, the advancement of scientific research, and accompanying governmental administrative costs. There is little doubt that this trend will continue. As the proportion of public spending on personal health care increases, there are parallel demands for greater controls.

When viewing selected components of medical care delivery, hospital room costs represent the most rapid growth rates in the United States. Medical care costs have consistently outpaced price increases for just about all other consumer goods and services over the past several decades. Even with this rate of growth the daily charge rate for a semiprivate room in a hospital has increased much more rapidly than medical care prices in general (see Figure 111). From 1958 to

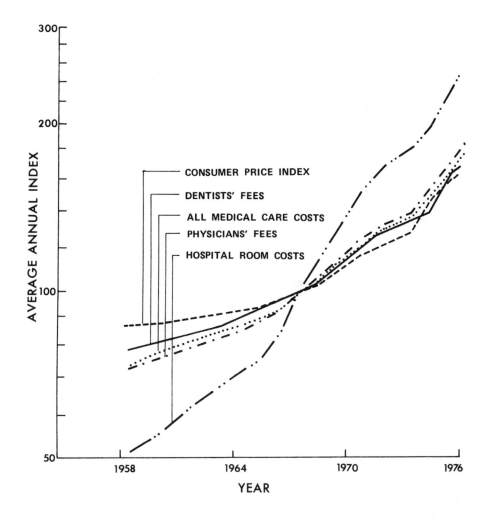

Source: Bureau of Labor Statistics

Fig. 111. Rising health care costs in the United States from 1958 to 1976.

1976, for example, physicians' fees, dentists' fees, and all medical care costs have more or less followed the rising consumer price index. Again, hospital room charges are the exception. Many factors have contributed to this rapid increase. Included are improvements in medical technologies, applications of new procedures and techniques, increasing numbers of hospital personnel, a rapidly rising wage rate for hospital employees, and increasingly more services demanded on the part of patients. The latter phenomenon is partly related to increases in health care coverage programs resulting from collective bargaining, competitive increases in fringe benefits, and more government expenditures.

This brief exposition of some of the factors contributing to the economic crisis in health care can be equated with the tip of an iceberg. An ample literature in health care economics exists as part of an area of study and application peripherally associated with medical geography. The medical geographer engaged in health care delivery planning will quickly develop an appreciation of the need to incorporate aspects of medical economics in the development of long-term goals. Aspects of the economics of health care have been incorporated into formal federal and state programmatical health planning practice. Public reaction to increased health care costs has been channeled through Health Systems Agencies that often manifest a bureaucratic response to the health care industry. This has resulted in forms of conflict.

The Bureaucratic Response and Conflicts

Many interests are obviously involved in health care delivery. As already mentioned, thre is a general tendency to broadly divide these interests into providers of health care and consumers of health care. This distinction can be taken to task in many ways. The National Health Planning and Resources Development Act of 1974 makes it clear that providers of health care cannot control health planning agencies and that a majority of representation on the boards should be from consumers. But there are many grey areas. Should a large industry paying most, if not all, of the health care costs of its employees be considered a provider or a consumer? Is a Health Systems Agency, as defined by the recent legislation, a provider or consumer group? Part of our nation's increased cost for the delivery of health care includes the operational budgets of more than 200 Health Systems Agencies. In practice, there is little doubt that the intent of health planning agencies is in the interest of consumers of health care. Officially recognized health planning agencies now have more authority than ever to control and contain providers of health care. Many providers of health care are attempting to cling to the free enterprise traditions that gave initial impetus to the growth of the health care industry of the United States. With hospital proposals as actions and Health Systems Agencies' reviews as reactions, conflict has become institutionalized. Part of the problem, many providers claim, is the bureaucratic response of health planning agencies. In support of this allegation of bureaucratic behavior they offer the complicated review process as an example. Conversely, many health planners contend that such a process is necessary because of provider reactions, especially in finding "loopholes" or other methods of bypassing formalized health planning policies to attain particular ends.

The review process is indeed complicated. The 1974 health planning legislation can be considered a major reorganization of federally supported health planning at all levels within the country. In many locales it was necessary to create new agencies. The newly defined agencies are responsible for many more aspects of health care planning than ever before, with a clearcut mandate to help control the rapid increases in health care costs.

Several kinds of agencies were created and different responsibilities have been assigned. Agency interrelationships have been carefully explained in a recent publication of the Midwest Center for Health Planning.[46] Reference to Figure 112, a flow chart of the various elements of the health planning process, assists in understanding these relationships. The following nomenclature is essential to understanding these processes (see Appendix A for further details). Within this context, "Secretary" refers to the Secretary of the Department of Health, Education, and Welfare. SHPDA refers to State Health Planning and Development Agencies. The SHCC (Statewide Health Coordinating Council) is a citizen council comprised primarily of consumers. The local HSA may be either private, nonprofit, or public, and has broad reaching review responsibilities in defined local health service areas. Responsibilities of the HSA include the development of a Health Goals Plan (HSP) and a more short-range priorities plan (AIP).

Figure 107 indicates 10 paths of agency interaction. Each path is concerned with a specialized function. The first path deals with the approval or disapproval of forms of federal spending or other methods of financial involvement. Included are just about all funds proposed to be used by providers under the Public Health Service Act. They include community mental health, alcoholism programs and many others. Initially a community agency or institution applies for funds through the Health Systems Agency. The Health Systems Agency reviews and approves or disapproves the application. It then moves to the Secretary of DHEW for similar action. The simplest solution is that if the project is approved at those two levels it is normally funded. If the HSA disapproves and the Secretary approves, the matter is turned over the the SHPDA. The annual budget of each HSA also needs approval at state and national levels, as indicated by the second path in Figure 112. A plan must be included with the budget submission. The third path shows the process HSA's must follow for establishing an area health services development fund. The application for establishing such a fund is submitted by the HSA to the state level coordinating council. It is then passed on to the Secretary with comments. If successfully reviewed by the Secretary, it is returned to the HSA. Once the area health services development fund has been approved, community agencies or organizations can apply for funds through the Health Systems Agency. An approval or disapproval is subsequently returned to the local agency requesting funds.

The flow process at the state level is indicated by paths 5 and 6. The fifth path shows the process required in developing a State Health Plan (SHP). The intent is to merge all local Health Systems Agency plans into the final plan for an entire state. Health Systems Agencies send plans to the State Health Planning

AGENCY RELATIONSHIPS

Under P. L. 93 — 641

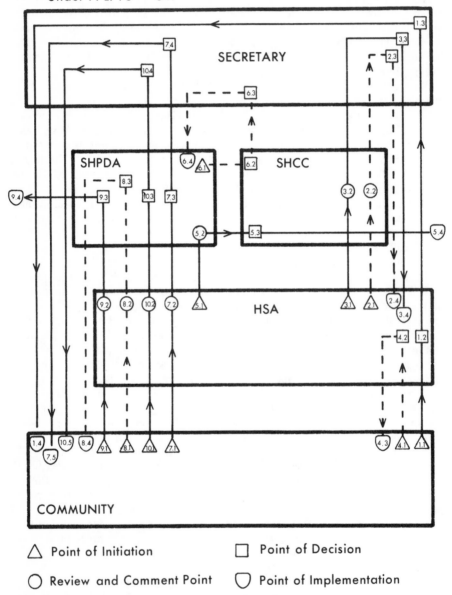

Fig. 112. Agency relationships under the Health Planning and Development Act of 1974 (P.L. 93-641). Ten paths have been identified.

and Development Agency (SHPDA). The latter agency integrates these plans into a larger document suited for coordinating statewide needs. The material is then forwarded to the SHCC for final approval. A state plan is then released to the public. The SHPDA is also responsible for devising development review and approval cycles for state plans under federal programs. Shown in path six, the SHPDA initially submits such plans to the SHCC. They are then forwarded to the Secretary for action. If approved, they are returned to the SHPDA.

The next four processes are various forms of review. The linkages indicated as path 7 pertain to institutions eligible under the Social Security Act. An institution with a proposed capital expenditure project submits a proposal to the SHPDA through the local HSA. In many instances this is done simultaneously. The HSA is empowered to review and comment. Final approval, however, rests with the statewide agency. An approved project is sent to the Secretary for reimbursement of projects. The secretary then deals with the institution proposing the expenditure. The eighth channel varies from state to state. Highest approval is at the statewide level, but national standards must be met. Any institution with a project requiring a state Certificate of Need submits a proposal to the local agency with the option of sending the proposal to the state agency at the same time. Actions are recommended to the state by local agencies and the state has the authority to approve or disapprove the application. Approved applications are granted the required Certificate of Need (see Appendix A).

The ninth path, still somewhat nebulous, pertains to "appropriateness" of virtually all health services offered within any given state. To obtain an appropriateness review, local agencies first supply necessary information to local HSA's. The HSA's in turn review the material and recommend action to the SHPDA. The SHPDA then makes a decision pertaining to appropriateness and subsequently publicizes the information. The tenth review pathway is one of the most important because it applies to any application for federal assistance for medical facilities construction programs. In effect, this part of the program offers more coordinated controls intended to integrate any new construction with overall health care activities within regions. Institutions requesting such support apply first to local HSA's. After review the local agency forwards proposals to the SHPDA. Public institutions may bypass the statewide agency in many instances. If the applications reach the state level and are approved, they are forwarded to the Secretary for further review. New developments must be in accord with overall State Medical Facilities Plans. Favorable review at the Secretarial level means that, given available funds, the projects can proceed.

"Appropriateness" has not been well defined, and there has been scant specific national level guidance pertaining to what appropriateness review actually means. In May, 1978, a notice of proposed rule making was published in the *Federal Register.*[47] A concise definition was put forth: "Appropriateness means a finding that a service meets the needs of a population in accordance with criteria adopted by the review agency." Criteria have been established, and they pertain to the well known concepts in health planning of acceptability, accessability, availability, continuity, cost, and quality. In order to avoid the possibility of some local disagreements, a check and balance system exists because local and statewide agencies work jointly on appropriateness reviews. This review requires an analysis of existing institutional health services, and any new services proposed must concur with Certificate of Need programs. A two-year time span can be involved because services offered by an institution twelve months prior to the review, as well as those proposed for the 12 months following the review, are taken into consideration. This provision makes it extremely difficult for an institution to suspend services temporarily in an attempt to avoid the review process.

As with any new program, the 1974 health planning legislation will not be easy to implement. It requires added inputs of federal funds in the face of accelerating health care costs. It virtually forces health care providers into taking part in coordinated health planning policy, but has substantially diminished provider input at the local level of health planning. Frankenhoff has suggested several barriers to the implementation of this program.[48] They include:

1. Except during periods of national emergency the United States does not have a traditional national health planning structure.
2. Past health planning programs have not been successful in terms of coordinated planning.
3. Acceptance of health planning at the local level will be difficult because people generally relate health planning to actual physical health care delivery mechanisms as proposed to intangible planning programs.
4. There is a political jurisdiction problem. While Health Systems Agencies were established with SMSA's in mind, it was also necessary to exhaust the country using the counties as building blocks to demarcate planning areas (see Figure 98).
5. Health Systems Agencies are not totally accountable to state and local government.
6. Levels of operational funding for HSA's are too low.
7. Provider groups view the new program as a threat to the varying degrees of independence they have traditionally enjoyed in the provision of health services.
8. There is inadequate health planning manpower to carry out the necessary programs.

These barriers contribute to a somewhat unique planning environment, and according to Frankenhoff, HSA's will have to develop strategies for intervention. This can best be accomplished through programs incorporating the cooperation of community, state, and federal agencies involved with health care and other forms of urban and regional planning agencies.

A REDEFINED ROLE FOR THE MEDICAL GEOGRAPHER IN HEALTH PLANNING

From 1946 to 1966, proportionately few professional geographers were engaged in health planning on a regular basis. While important contributions were made in the area of allocation modeling and service area definition methodologies, the less than comprehensive nature of the health planning environment during those two decades did not require the kinds of geographical information specified by the act of 1974. As so well stated by Frankenhoff, there is an acute manpower shortage in health planning. In addition, substantial geographical information is now required as part of the intended trend toward more comprehensive planning. When considering the topics of the various chapters in this book, there is a definite need for most of the tasks that medical geographers are equipped to accomplish. The determination of spatial variations utilizing different morbidity and mortality rates and ratios can lead to regional mosaics of health status through various methods of disease mapping. Knowledge of environmental risk factors in operation can offer much in the way of understanding environmental risk factors, and this kind of information is required under the new legislation. Aspects of disease diffusion also pertain to an even larger set of risk factors that can be measured. Geographical studies of associative factors can produce meaningful information about the health status of HSA populations. Measures of distributions of health care resources and facilities in relation to availability and accessibility can be accomplished through some of the methodologies identified in this chapter as well as others not considered here.

The most numerous opportunities for medical geographers to work for or with health planning agencies are at the local level. One of the best combinations of skills the geographer has to offer consists of methodologies for the collection, organization, and analysis of information made available on the basis of small subareas within the larger Health Systems Areas. These kinds of data requirements are spelled out quite clearly in recent health planning information handbooks published by the Department of Health, Education, and Welfare.[49]

Since SMSA's were given consideration in the formation of the Health Service Areas shown within Figure 98, an excellent mechanism for accomplishing the necessary data handling already exists in several hundred metropolitan areas of the United States. This tool that can be extremely important in the various processes involved in health planning is in the form of geographic base files, normally developed in conjunction with the U.S. Bureau of the Census. These files have been under development for nearly a decade, and very early during this period Levy was quick to point out the utility of using these files in the development of integrated health information systems.[50] Figure 113 illustrates the overall model suggested by Levy and utilized in Kansas City, Missouri for the development of a health information system. While Levy's system pertains to the Kansas City Health Department, it is constructed in such a manner as to be appropriate to the data needs of Health Systems Agencies as set forth by the Department of Health, Education, and Welfare. His model includes financial, socioeconomic, resource, hospital inpatient and outpatient, ambulatory care, assessment of quality care, and a variety of other information inputs to the overall collection procedure. Incorporated in Levy's model is the use of a geographic base file. The development of programs geared toward the use of these files is a natural direction for the medical geographer to follow. In addition, the use of such a methodology by a Health Systems Agency could do

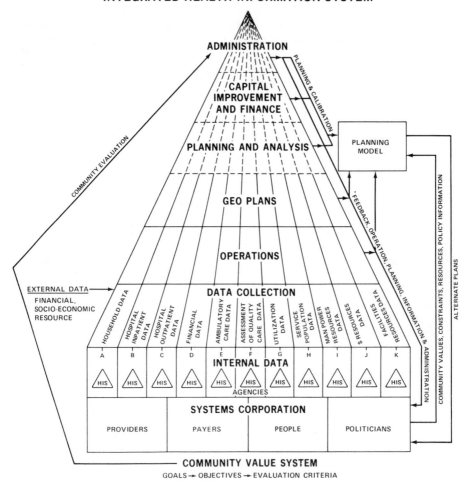

Fig. 113. Levy's interpretation of the Kansas City Integrated Health Information System.

much to alleviate Frankenhoff's barrier pertaining to cooperation with other planning agencies in regions. Geographic base files are discussed in more detail in Chapter 8.

NOTES

[1] Andrew Learmonth. *Patterns of Disease and Hunger: A Study in Medical Geography.* London: David and Charles (1978), pp. 210-241.

[2] Milton I. Roemer. *Systems of Health Care.* New York: Springer (1977).

[3] Stephen J. Kunitz and Andrew A. Sorensen. "The Effects of Regional Planning on a Rural Hospital: A Case Study," *Social Science and Medicine (Medical Geography),* forthcoming, 1979.

[4] Gary W. Shannon and G. E. Alan Dever. *Health Care Delivery: Spatial Perspectives.* New York: McGraw-Hill (1974).

[5] Commission on Hospital Care. *Hospital Care in the United States.* New York: The Commonwealth Fund (1974).

[6] J. Joel May. *Health Planning: Its Past and Potential.* Health Administration Perspectives No. 5. Chicago: Center for Health Administration (1967).

[7] Leslie Morgan Abee and Anna Mae Baney. *The Nation's Health Facilities: Ten Years of Hill-Burton Hospital and Medical Facilities Program, 1946-1956.* Washington: U.S. Department of Health, Education, and Welfare, Public Health Service (1958), p. 11.

[8] Commission on Hospital Care, op. cit.

[9] J. Joel May, op. cit.

[10] Monroe Lerner and Odin W. Anderson. *Health Progress in the United States 1900-1960.* Chicago: University of Chicago Press (1963).

[11] Gerald F. Pyle. *Heart Disease, Cancer and Stroke in Chicago: A Geographical Analysis with Facilities Plans for 1980.* Chicago: University of Chicago, Department of Geography Research Monograph 134 (1971).

[12] Joseph W. Mountin, Emily K. Hankla, and George B. Druzina. *Ten Years of Federal Grants-in-Aid for Public Health, 1936-1946.* Public Health Service Bulletin No. 300, Washington, D.C., 1946.

[13] Alan E. Treloar and Don Chill. *Patient Care Facilities: Construction Needs and Hill-Burton Accomplishments.* Hospital Monograph Series No. 10. Chicago: American Hospital Association (1961), Chap. 2.

[14] "Areawide Planning for Hospitals and Related Health Facilities," a report of the Joint Committee of the American Hospital Association and the Public Health Service, U.S. Department of Health, Education, and Welfare, Public Health Service, Publication No. 885. Washington: U.S. Government Printing Office (1961).

[15] Dwight L. Wilbur. "Quality and Availability of Care Under Regional Medical Programs," *Journal of the American Medical Association,* March 11, 1968, pp. 143-47.

[16] Adapted from "Health Systems Plan" Vol. 1 (Data Analysis), Health Planning and Development Council, Wooster, Ohio (March, 1978).

[17] *Federal Register.* "Health Systems Agencies: Designation and Funding," Department of Health, Education, and Welfare, Public Health Service (March 26, 1976).

[18] "Geographic Variation: Measures of Health, Utilization, Resources, and Expenditures," *Health, United States 1976-1977.* Washington: U.S. Department of Health, Education, and Welfare, Health Resources Administration (1978), pp. 43-60.

[19] Gary W. Shannon and G. E. Alan Dever, op. cit., pp. 8-35.

[20] S. Godlund. "Population, Regional Hospitals, Transportation Facilities and Regions: Planning the Location of Regional Hospitals in Sweden," *Lund Studies in Geography*, No. 21. Lund, Sweden: Gleerup (1961). William L. Garrison et al. *Studies of Highway Development and Geographic Change*. Seattle: University of Washington Press (1959).

[21] Gary W. Shannon, Rashid L. Bashshur, and Charles Metzner. "The Concept of Distance as a Factor in Accessibility and Utilization of Health Care," *Medical Care Review*, Vol. 26 (1969), pp. 143-161.

[22] Robert Earickson. *The Spatial Behavior of Hospital Patients*. Chicago: University of Chicago, Department of Geography, Research Monograph No. 124 (1970).

[23] Richard L. Morrill and Robert J. Earickson. "Hospital Variation and Patient Travel Distances," *Inquiry*, Vol. 5 (1968), pp. 1-9.

[24] Gerald F. Pyle and Bruce M. Lauer. "Comparing Spatial Configurations: Hospital Service Areas and Disease Rates," *Economic Geography*, Vol. 51 (1975), pp. 50-68.

[25] C. E. Bell and D. A. Nen. "Optimal Planning of an Emergency Ambulance Service," *Socio-Economic Planning Sciences*, Vol. 3 (1969), pp. 95-101.

[26] Richard L. Morrill and Robert J. Earickson. "Variation in the Use and Character of Chicago Area Hospitals," *Health Services Research*, Vol. 3 (1968), pp. 224-238.

[27] "Patient Origin Study," Seven County Health Planning Council, Wooster, Ohio (1973).

[28] Gerald F. Pyle and Bruce M. Lauer, op. cit.

[29] G. W. Shannon and C. W. Spurlock, "Urban Ecological Containers, Environmental Risk Cells, and the Use of Medical Services," *Economic Geography*, Vol. 52 (1976), pp. 171-180.

[30] D. Lefever. "Measuring Geographical Concentration by Means of the Standard Deviational Ellipse," *American Journal of Sociology*, Vol. 32 (1926), pp. 88-94.

[31] Gary W. Shannon. "Space, Time and Illness Behavior," *Social Science and Medicine (Medical Geography)*, Vol. 11 (November, 1977), pp. 683-689.

[32] Horatio Fabrega, Jr. *Disease and Social Behavior: An Interdisciplinary Perspective.* Cambridge, Mass.: MIT Press (1974).

[33] "Advances in Health Survey Methods" and "Experiments in Interviewing Techniques: Field Experiments in Health Reporting, 1971-1977," National Center for Health Services Research, U.S. Department of Health, Education, and Welfare, Public Health Service, Health Resources Administration. Washington: DHEW Publication No. (HCA)77-3154 and (HCA)78-3204 (1977 and 1978).

[34] Pierre deVise. "Physician Migration from Inland to Coastal States: Antipodal Example of Illinois and California," *Journal of Medical Education*, Vol. 48 (1973), pp. 141-151.

[35] Gary W. Shannon and G. E. Alan Dever, op. cit., pp. 70-88.

[36] Donald Dewey. *Where the Doctors Have Gone.* Chicago: Illinois Regional Medical Program (1973).

[37] Jerome W. Lubin et al. "How Distance Affects Physician Activity," *The Modern Hospital*, July, 1966.

[38] Saul F. Rosenthal. "Target Populations and Physician Populations: The Effects of Density and Change," *Social Science and Medicine (Medical Geography)*, Vol. 12 (1978), pp. 111-115.

[39] See Herbert Harvey Hyman. *Health Planning: A Systematic Approach.* Germantown, Maryland: Aspen Systems Corporation (1975) and Ruth Roemer, Charles Kramer, and Jeanne E. Fink. *Planning Urban Health Services: From Jungle to System.* New York: Springer (1975).

[40] Gerald F. Pyle and Gary F. Stein. "Some Spatial Implications of Health Maintenance Organizations," paper presented to the Association of American Geographers, Atlanta, Georgia (1973).

[41] David A. Gee. "Ambulatory Care," *Hospitals*, Vol. 44 (1970), p. 73.

[42] E. L. Crosby. "Hospitals as the Center of the Health Care Universe," *Hospitals,* January 1, 1970, p. 52.

[43] Gerald F. Pyle, op. cit., pp. 157–200.

[44] "Geographic Variation: Measures of Health, Utilization, Resources, and Expenditures," *Health, United States 1976-1977,* op. cit., pp. 341–395.

[45] "Health, United States, 1976-1977: Chartbook," U.S. Department of Health, Education, and Welfare, Public Health Service. Washington: DHEW Publication No. (HRA)77-1233 (1977).

[46] "Agency Relationships Under P. L. 93-641: A Chartbook." Midwest Center for Health Planning, Madison, Wisconsin (1978).

[47] "Review of Appropriateness: Analysis of Proposed Rules." Midwest Center for Health Planning, Madison, Wisconsin (1978).

[48] Charles A. Frankenhoff. "The Planning Environment of Health Systems Agencies," *Inquiry,* Vol. 14 (1977), pp. 217–228.

[49] "A Guide to the Development of Health Resource Inventories" and "A Data Acquisition and Analysis Handbook for Health Planners." U.S. Department of Health, Education, and Welfare, Public Health Service, Health Resources Administration. Washington: DHEW Publication Nos. (HRA)77-14506 and (HRA)77-14506.

[50] Richard M. Levy. "Use of a Geographic Base File in a Health Information System." U.S. Department of Commerce, Bureau of the Census. Washington: Computerized Geographic Coding Series GE 60 No. 3 (1972).

Chapter 8

APPLICATIONS OF GEOCODING SYSTEMS IN MEDICAL GEOGRAPHY

The recommendation in the previous chapter that Health Systems Agencies in the United States and similar authorities in other countries adopt integrated health information systems modeled after the Kansas City operation is predicated on the assumption that specific geographic areas have a functioning geographic base file. These files are based on computerized mapping systems. In some countries, the United Kingdom for example, the Ordinance Survey has attained accurate urban detail by encoding at the parcel level within blocks.[1] While many engineering mapping systems have been developed over the years in various locations in the United States, there has been no overall national effort to organize a unified mapping and information retrieval system until quite recently. The efforts of the U.S. Bureau of Census in the development of local geographic base files offers a promising beginning. During the late 1960s and early 1970s, the Bureau of Census initiated an effort to construct computerized geographic base files in the most urbanized parts of the United States for purposes of eventual automated enumeration. There are now approximately 300 such files known as DIME (Dual Independent Map Encoding) Files.

THE THEORETICAL BASIS

DIME Files are based on dual planar surfaces.[2] In this dual structure, two independent matrices are utilized. One is a set of line boundaries and the second is a network of areas. The Dual Independent Map Encoding takes place when the basic file is created by encoding the nodes connecting line segments on the one network and areas enclosed by the nodes and line segments on the second (see Figure 114). The combined network is represented within an encoded file and all land area is accounted for. With the addition of geographic coordinates it is possible to use a computer to completely replicate the source information.

Vertices, Lines, and Enclosed Areas

The DIME system is actually a geographic dictionary combining linear graphics and alphanumeric information. The planar structure contains implicitly defined sets of distinguishing points. This is accomplished by algorithmic recognition. The DIME dictionaries contain sets of linear graphs with alphanumeric names attached to three types of elements defining the graphs.[3] These three elements are vertices, lines, and encoded areas. When encoded they form separate incidence matrices: line segment—node, line segment—enclosed area, and enclosed area—node. In less abstract terms, these elements contained within DIME Files are street segments (Lines), nodes indicating the intersection of streets (Vertices) and city blocks (Enclosed areas). This relationship is depicted within Figure 115. A functioning DIME File is composed of segment records defined as lengths of streets or other features between two specific nodes or vertices. In addition to such manmade geographic features as street networks, physiographic features

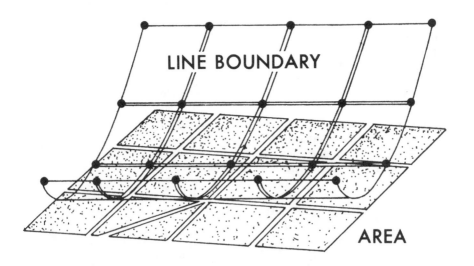

Fig. 114. The derivation of "Dual" in DIME Systems.

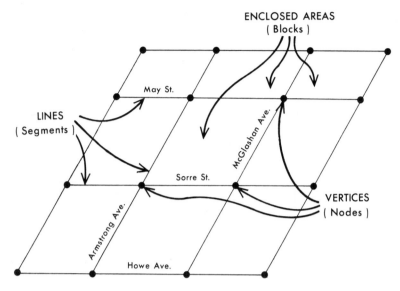

Fig. 115. A diagrammatic explanation of lines, enclosed areas and vertices in DIME systems.

(i.e., rivers, shorelines, canals, and lakes) are also included within DIME systems. Imaginary lines defining political and other kinds of boundaries are also incorporated.

A process termed "chaining" is essential to the proper operation of DIME Files. One method of chaining is based on nodes with associated segment codes arranged in a cyclic fashion allowing for the identification of specific areas on the basis of an encircled path. A second method chains areas around nodes. The process of chaining a string of segments that bound a block is shown within Figure 116. This elementary illustration explains how the computer reads from one node to another. Beginning with node 31 at the intersection of May Street and Armstrong Avenue, the computer reads to node 32 at the intersection of McGlashan Avenue and May street. The process of chaining then begins by reading from node 32 to node 33, the intersection of Sorre Street and McGlashan Avenue. The process continues from node 33 to node 34, back to node 31 to enclose block number 105. Left and right blocks are included in the DIME system on a from node to node basis. With this example of chaining the right block is always 105. Included within the DIME system are ranges of numeric addresses sequenced from lowest to highest along street segments corresponding with left and right sides of each street segment. DIME Files become alphanumeric geographic dictionaries when all known low to high address

Segment Name	From Node	To Node	Block Left	Block Right
May St	31 ——→ 32		102	105
McGlashan Ave	32 ⇇ ⟹ 33		104	105
Sorre St	33 ⇇ ⟹ 34		108	105
Armstrong Ave	34 ⇇ —→ 31		106	105

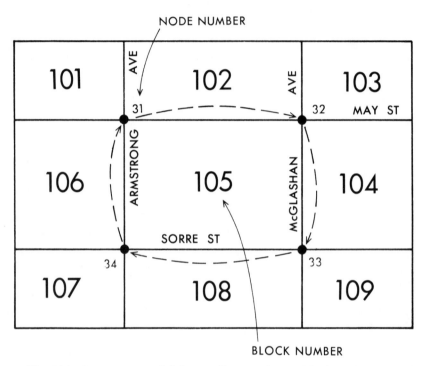

Fig. 116. One process of "chaining" to enclose a block within a DIME system.

ranges for all segments from one node to the next are stored as computerized records. The size of an actual DIME File varies with the size of a metropolitan area. A DIME encoded area with about 800,000 people will have a file of approximately 50,000 records, while a large metropolitan area of 6,000,000 persons may have from 350,000 to 400,000 records, depending upon progress in encoding information and the extent of the settled area incorporated. In many metropolitan areas DIME Files have not yet been completed. As the 1980 census is approached in the United States, DIME Files will be used to the extent that it is possible. For applications in medical geography DIME Files mean even more than the enumeration essential to a working population base. They are a necessary ingredient to optimal handling of health information.

The Matching Process

The capability of matching records from more than one file with address ranges is a valuable feature of DIME Files. The census use study of the U.S. Bureau of Census has developed two programs for matching information, ADMATCH and UNIMATCH.[4] Since ADMATCH systems (these systems include more than one single program) are the most widely used, that process is explained here. With the ADMATCH system it is necessary to have a reference file (DIME) and a data file. A three-phase operation takes place. The first consists of preprocessing. In this operation a preprocessor program determines addresses and creates a character match key. This phase includes city, state, and other geographic codes as well as standardized street names. The data file, local health information for example, and reference file are then sorted on geographic information in the match key, including postal zip codes, geographic place information, street names, and house numbers or address ranges. The second ADMATCH program matches by comparing items in the match keys of the data file and the reference file. Successful matches are then placed into a matched file through a third, or post-processor step. If successful matches do not occur for one reason or another, there are several automated and some manual methods to reach an eventual match.

The matching process and subsequent results are shown within Figure 117. Given a local health data file consisting of street names and addresses of patients or victims and pertinent geographic information pertaining to place of residence, health-related data such a diagnosis, treatment, age, sex, etc., can also be included. The local health data file is then matched with the DIME reference file resulting in an address matched health data file. The new file contains a combination of the information from the other two, and this results in a stored listing of street names and numbers, census blocks and tracts, and other pertinent geographic entities. The other geographic entities might include information added to the reference file pertaining to health planning districts. The file of aggregated geographic data can then be programmed to print tabulations of aggregated geographic information, including numbers of cases, victims or patients, by census blocks in tabulated form. The user of the information can also opt to link the file of aggregated geographic data with various ongoing systems of computer maps.

SOME RECOMMENDED APPLICATIONS IN
MEDICAL GEOGRAPHY

The value of DIME Files in medical geography cannot be underemphasized. It is possible to use DIME Files to accomplish most of the approaches and methods

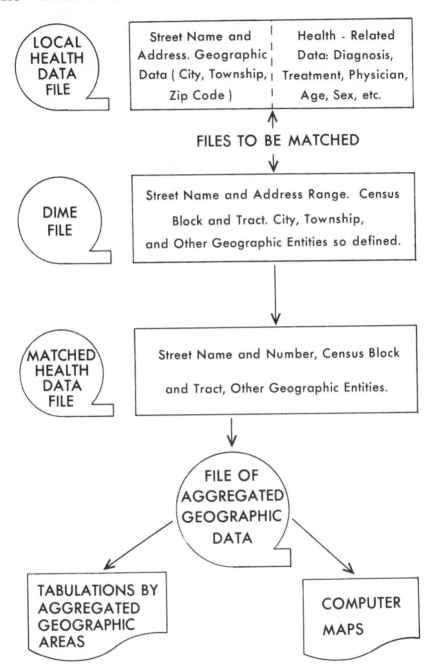

Fig. 117. A schematic representation of using a geographic base file with a local health information system.

discussed with Chapters 2 through 7 of this book. With an up-to-date population base enumerating numbers of inhabitants by enclosed areas, it is possible to rapidly and efficiently compute a wide variety of disease and illness rates and ratios. In the area of disease mapping, particularly with the increased use of automated cartography, DIME Files become a logical and sometimes necessary ingredient. By locating victims of infectious diseases it is possible to determine ecological correlates in the area of environmental health planning. It would be possible with the use of DIME Files to actually build temporal sequences of disease reporting and formulate a more detailed understanding of the process of disease diffusion. In terms of associative and statistical research the use of DIME Files could increase our knowledge ten-fold. In the area of health care planning DIME Files are already being used in many urban locations within the United States. More widespread use of these files appears to be restricted primarily because of either local politics or the lack of coordinated efforts leading to integrated health information systems. Clearly, while a major work could, and probably has been, developed pertaining to the use of geographic base files in the area of health care, the examples offered below pertain to limited applications using the Akron, Ohio SMSA DIME File.

Automated Mapping with a Geocoding System

If automated mapping methods are to be merged with geographic base files, it is necessary at the onset to append geographic coordinates to nodes or vertices. Having accomplished the insertion of coordinates, the incorporation of automated mapping is a simple step in systems development. This kind of operation is outlined within Figure 118. Initially, ADMATCHed information is selected to be mapped and the actual automated mapping program is determined. The DIME File is affixed with coordinates and the data file is merged with those coordinates. Once the coordinates are attached to the data file it is a matter of scaling the data file in a predetermined method, or perhaps several methods, as input to the mapping program. Class intervals and various mapping options are then selected, and the map is produced as computer output.

Making use of the completed and operational Akron DIME File and reported prevalence of confirmed cases of viral encephalitis in Akron from 1965 to 1976, Figures 119 through 122 have been produced as examples of automated mapping with ADMATCHed information. Figure 119 shows class intervals based on standard deviations of the actual numbers of reported cases of viral encephalitis within the city. While ranges of numbers are given in relation to class intervals, such a map merely shows a count of cases with no standardization. Age-adjusted rates for the population under 18 years of age are shown within Figure 120. Some meaningful comparisons can be made from this cartographic pattern because of the age standardization. The visual impression of concentrations of cases is apparent. It is also possible to standardize by area as shown within Figure 121. In this instance class intervals are determined as a ratio of cases per acre within census tracts. The cartographic pattern has changed somewhat, and shows that when standardizing by area is accomplished the researcher is offered an alternative in attempting to identify concentrations of higher rates.

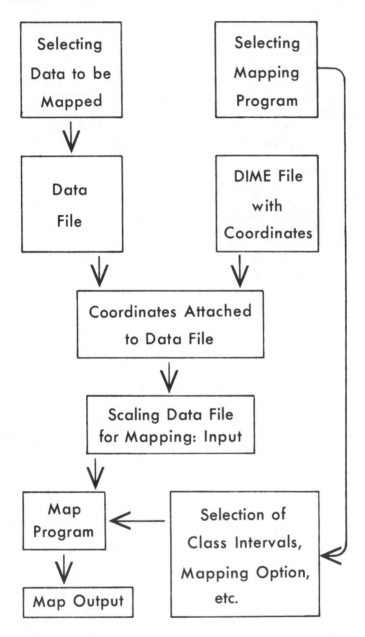

Fig. 118. A diagrammatic representation of computer graphics in relation to DIME files.

ENCEPHALITIS

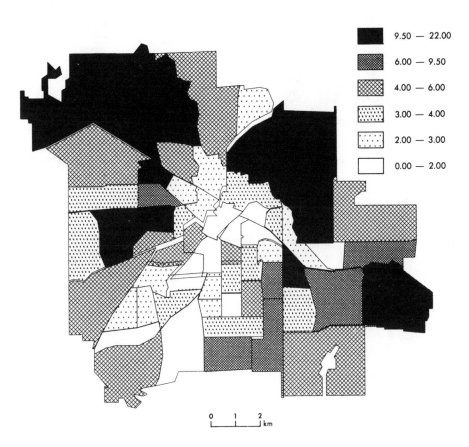

Fig. 119. The distribution of Encephalitis in Akron, Ohio in the 1970s. This map was developed with the assistance of the Akron DIME File.

ENCEPHALITIS RATES PER POPULATION

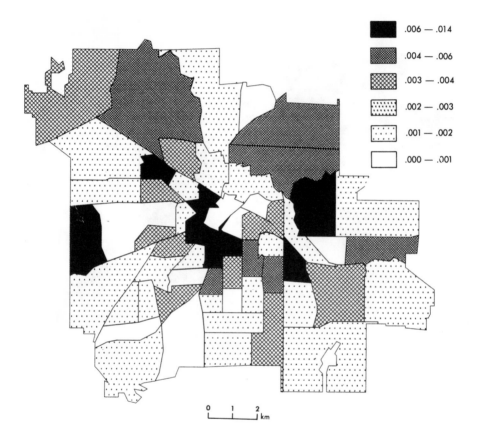

Fig. 120. Encephalitis rates in Akron in relation to population under 18 years of age.

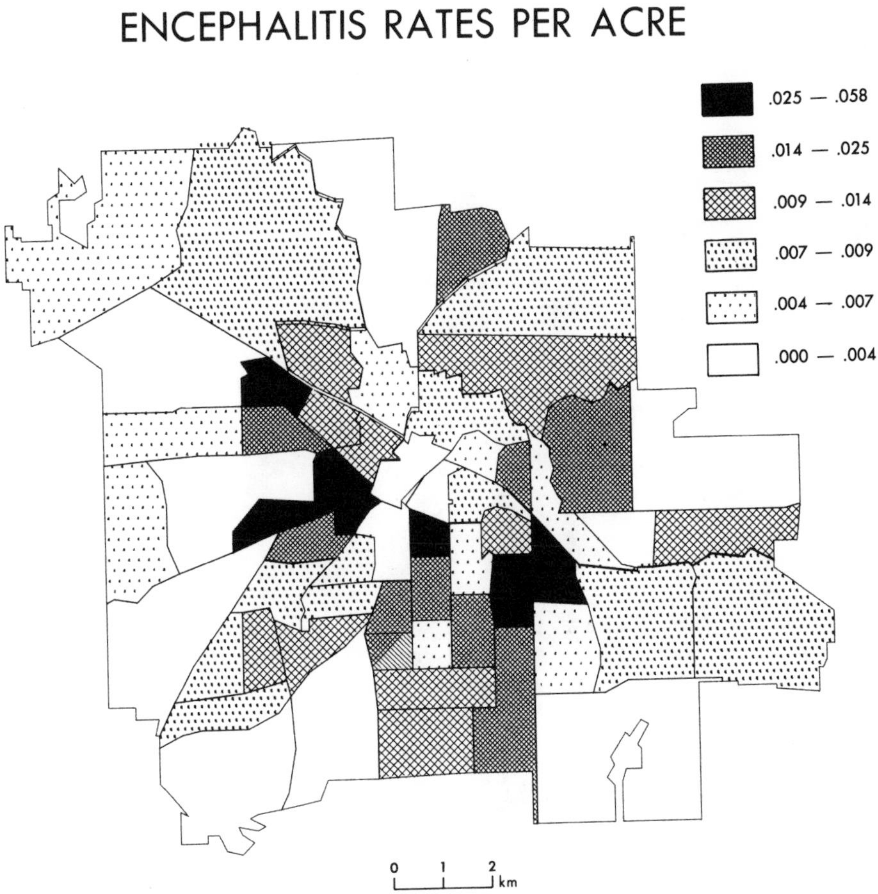
ENCEPHALITIS RATES PER ACRE
.025 — .058
.014 — .025
.009 — .014
.007 — .009
.004 — .007
.000 — .004
0 1 2
km

Fig. 121. Encephalitis rates per acre in Akron, Ohio.

Linkages of geographic base files to automated mapping systems consists of much more than the structuring of these simple choroplethic maps. Given the information stored within the Akron DIME File it is possible to plot a complete street pattern of the city and overlay specific locations of the encephalitis cases (see Figure 122). Medical geography researchers preferring dot maps have the capability through the use of DIME Files to plot cases in such a manner. With the addition of the Akron drainage pattern it is possible to gain the visual

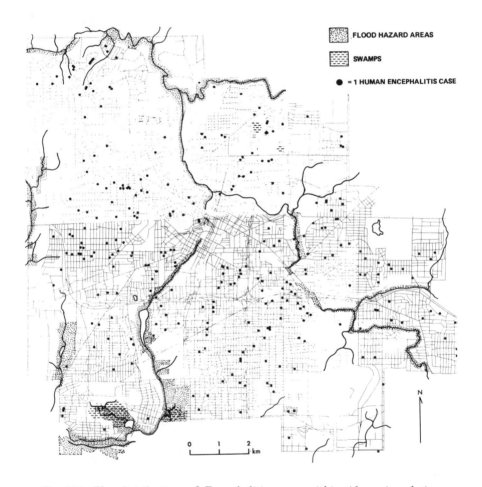

Fig. 122. The distribution of Encephalitis cases within Akron in relation to the drainage system. The underlying base map was developed from the Akron DIME File, and the actual cases were located automatically with the geocoding system.

impression of some concentrations of encephalitis cases either close to poorly drained areas or to floodplains.

Using a DIME File for Planning Emergency Medical Services

DIME Files are already in use in some major cities in the United States for purposes of planning the improvement of the delivery of Emergency Medical Services. Efforts were initiated in Akron in 1978 to use the DIME File for such a purpose. A sample Emergency Medical Services (EMS) data base was constructed by acquiring information for all emergency visits to Akron City Hospital during the month of July 1977. The file consisted of approximately 2,500 visits and included method of transportation, purpose of emergency room visit, and other pertinent information. The EMS file was matched with the Akron DIME File, and several different service areas were identified. One important issue pertained to the use of ambulances, both public and private, compared with private vehicles. Figures 123 and 124 include two contrasting service areas. The service area for those who used an ambulance to travel to the hospital is restricted primarily to the Akron central city area, with one large and several small pockets of intense travel to the hospital. By contrast, the service area of those using a private vehicle to travel to the hospital is quite extensive. A major concentration is still in the central city, where a third of the population resides, but there are areas of heavy use extending into most of suburban Summit County and the southwestern corner of Portage County. Other service areas were also identified by using the ADMATCHed information for major categories of health problems. Figure 125 shows the extent of the service area of Akron City Hospital within the two counties of the SMSA for trauma treatment, and Figure 126 shows a less extensive service area for cardiac patients. While a comprehensive EMS system has not yet been established for the Akron, Ohio area, the above kinds of inputs will prove to be useful when this is accomplished.

With such a DIME-related system, health care delivery planners can construct computer allocations of cases to EMS centers. In the forms of census and local health data, the actual DIME File and EMS use data can be used to model such an allocation system by sequentially examining the geographic base file, the network contained within the geographic base file, overall population distributions and the more specific distribution of proposed EMS centers (Figure 127). Many allocation models are available to accomplish this.[5] In an abstract sense, a DIME-related allocation model might function in a manner similar to that depicted within Figure 128. EMS Centers are located first on the basis of knowledge pertaining to need demonstrated by community use of various existing facilities. A DIME-determined network of major arterials is used to both plot EMS cases and determine the accessibility of major arterials. Areas radiating in terms of time and distance from specified centers can then be computed through several functioning algorithms to arrive at approximated travel thresholds for ambulances. As recently noted by Jon Mayer, time is absolutely critical in moving emergency victims to care centers.[6] A difference of from three to six minutes may result in the unnecessary loss of human life.

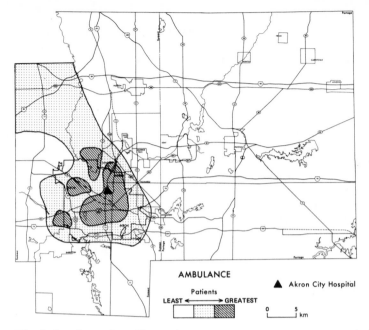

Fig. 123. Akron City Hospital emergancy patients using an ambulance as means of travel.

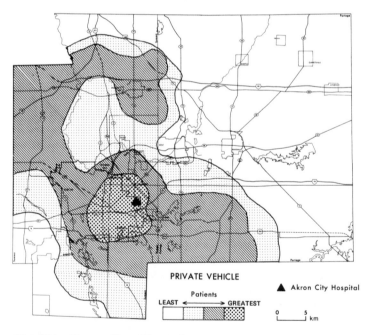

Fig. 124. Akron City Hospital emergency patients using a private vehicle to travel to the hospital.

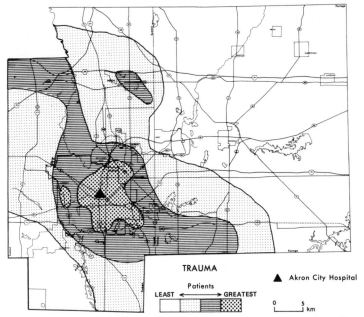

Fig. 125. The service area for emergency treatment for Trauma (Akron City Hospital).

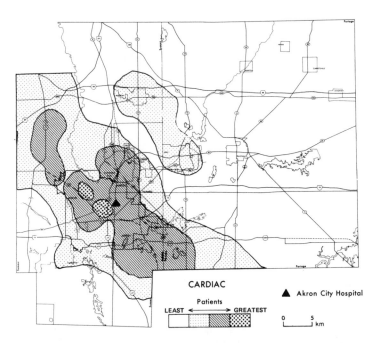

Fig. 126. The Akron City Hospital service area for those receiving emergency medical services for Cardiac problems.

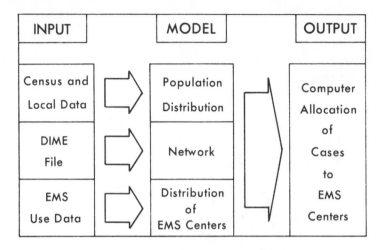

Fig. 127. A diagrammatic representation of use of a DIME file in the computer allocation of emergency patients to hospitals.

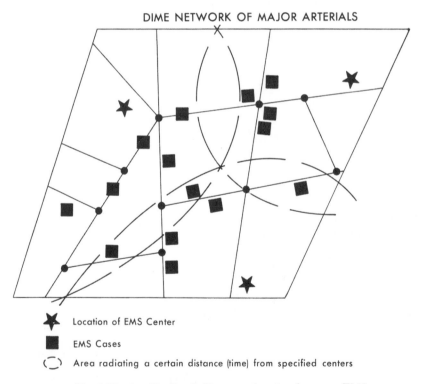

DIME NETWORK OF MAJOR ARTERIALS

★ Location of EMS Center

■ EMS Cases

◯ Area radiating a certain distance (time) from specified centers

Fig. 128. An idealized diagram showing how an EMS allocation model could function.

POSSIBLE FUTURE APPLICATIONS

This entire book has been about the geography of human life. The use of geographic base files by medical geographers in the form of information important to those delivering health care is an important short-term contribution. The improvement of reporting systems is a major long-term contribution. Problems of data reliability are a constant constraint in health care planning. As geographic base files in the standard form prescribed by the U.S. Bureau of Census are developed by more and more places, routine systems of reporting vital statistics can be greatly enhanced. With the improvement of mechanisms for retrieving should come increased use of reported information. Increased use of the information should hopefully result in more accurate reporting. If such information bases can be approved at local levels the type of information sent to state departments of health, and ultimately to federal agencies, can in turn be used to improve health status. Case studies of how this can be accomplished have been supported by the Bureau of Census.

NOTES

[1] James Corbett and George Farnsworth. "Theoretical Basis of Dual Independent Map Encoding." Conference Proceedings of the First International DIME Colloquium. U.S. Department of Commerce, Bureau of the Census. Washington: Census Use Study (1973).

[2] "Report No. 15, The Uses of GBF/DIME." U.S. Department of Commerce, Bureau of the Census. Washington: Census Use Study (1974).

[3] "Report No. 4, The DIME Geocoding System." U.S. Department of Commerce, Bureau of Census. Washington: Census Use Study (1970).

[4] Mathew A. Jaro. "OS ADMATCH." U.S. Department of Commerce, Bureau of Census. Washington: Census Use Study (1972). Also "ADMATCH Users Manual." U.S. Department of Commerce, Bureau of Census. Washington: Census Use Study (1970).

[5] Allen J. Scott. "Location–Allocation Systems: A Review," *Geographical Analysis,* Vol. 2 (1970), pp. 95–119.

[6] Jonathan D. Mayer. "Seattle's Paramedic Program: Geographical Distribution, Response Times, and Mortality," *Social Science and Medicine (Medical Geography),* forthcoming (1979).

APPENDIX A:
GLOSSARY OF HEALTH
PLANNING TERMS

ACCEPTABILITY—An overall assessment of the health care services that people receive.

ACCESSIBILITY—A measure of ability to obtain or use health care services, given they are available.

ACUTE CARE SERVICES—Intensive diagnostic treatment or restorative services used in providing treatment for illness or injury. Acute care services usually require short-term hospitalization generally not exceeding thirty days in length of stay.

ALLIED HEALTH PROFESSIONS—Specially trained and licensed (when necessary) health workers. Included as allied health professionals are dieticians, dental hygienists, physician assistants, etc. These workers are usually used to perform tasks ancillary to those of a physician.

AMBULATORY CARE—All types of health services that are provided on an out-patient basis. This term usually implies that the patient uses a location other than his home to receive services and departs the same day.

ANCILLARY HEALTH PERSONNEL—All health professionals excluding physicians, optometrists, pharmacists, podiatrists, and veterinarians.

ANNUAL IMPLEMENTATION PLAN (AIP)—A plan explaining how to implement short-term objectives leading toward more long-range goals of a health planning agency as detailed in its Health Systems Plan. All HSA's are required by P.L. 93-641 to develop an AIP.

AREA HEALTH EDUCATION CENTER (AHEC)—An organization or system of health, education, and service institutions having policies and programs frequently under the direction of a medical school or university health science center. The primary goals of these organizations are to improve the distribution, supply, quality, utilization, and efficiency of health personnel in relation to specific medically underserved areas. The primary objectives are to educate and train the health personnel specifically needed by that underserved community and to decentralize health manpower education, thereby increasing manpower supplies and providing a linkage between the health and education institutions in scarcity areas.

AVAILABILITY—A measure of the supply of health services and resources.

BLUE CROSS PLAN—A nonprofit, tax-exempt health service prepayment organizational structure providing coverage for health care and related services. A distinction should be made between individual plans and the national association (Blue Cross). Historically, the plans were largely the creation of the hospital industry, and designed to provide hospitals with a stable source of revenues, although formal association between Blue Cross and the American Hospital Association ended in 1972. A Blue Cross plan must be a nonprofit community service organization with a governing body including membership from a majority of public representives. Most plans are regulated by state insurance commissioners under special enabling legislation. Plans are exempt from federal income taxes and, in most states, from state taxes. Unlike most private insurance companies, the plans usually provide service rather than indemnity benefits, and often pay hospitals on the basis of reasonable costs as opposed to charges. There are approximately 70 plans in the United States.

BLUE SHIELD PLAN—A nonprofit, tax-exempt plan of a type originally established in 1939 which provides coverage for physicians' services. The individual plans should be distinguished from the National Association of Blue Shield Plans. Blue Shield coverage is commonly sold in conjunction with Blue Cross coverage, although this is not always the case. The relationship between Blue Cross and Blue Shield plans has been a cooperative one and it is not uncommon for the two organizations to have common boards and management. Blue Shield plans cover about 65 million Americans through their group and individual organizations. In addition, plan activities affect approximately 20 million persons through participation in various government programs, including Medicare (32 plans act as carriers under part B), Medicaid, and CHAMPUS. Most states have enacted special enabling legislation for Blue Shield Plans.

CERTIFICATE OF NEED—A certificate issued by a governmental body to an individual or organization proposing to construct or modify a health facility or offer a new or different health service. The intent of the certificate of need is that when a health care facility or service is available it is used by those for whom it is intended.

CHARACTERISTICS OF THE HEALTH SYSTEM—The major attributes of the health system that health planning agencies must consider in planning for the health system under P.L. 96-641. They include: cost, availability, accessibility, continuity, acceptability, and quality. When operational measures are applied to these characteristics they may be used to serve as indicators of health system performance. These six characteristics are a major component of the "Health System" taxonomy for planning under the 1974 legislation.

CLINIC—A facility, or part of one, for diagnosis and treatment of out-patients. Clinic is irregularly defined, sometimes either including or excluding physicians' offices. Some definitions of clinic are limited to facilities serving the medically indigent, and others are limited to medical education.

COMMUNITY HEALTH PROMOTION AND PROTECTION SERVICES—Those services directed at the community level toward improving the personal health behavior of residents and improving the quality of factors in the environment affecting human health. Included are:
- Health Education Services
- Environmental Quality Management
- Food Protection
- Occupational Health and Safety
- Radiation Safety
- Biomedical and Consumer Product Safety

COMMUNITY MENTAL HEALTH CENTER (CMHC)—An entity providing comprehensive (mostly ambulatory) mental health services primarily to individuals residing or employed in a defined catchment area. The term is defined in the Community Mental Health Centers Act (Section 201) which specifies the services to be provided and the requirements for the governance, organization and operation of the centers. The CMHC Act provides for federal financial assistance for the construction, development, and initial operation of CMHC's and, on an ongoing basis, for the cost of their consultation and education services.

CONSUMER—This is a technical term used in health planning legislation and programs usually applying to anyone who is not a provider of health care services. It is intended to include those who are not associated in any indirect or direct way with the provision of health care also.

DEPARTMENT OF HEALTH, EDUCATION, AND WELFARE (DHEW)—Created in 1953, a cabinet level department of the federal Executive Branch responsible for promoting and ensuring the highest level of health attainable for every individual and family in the United States; for the administration of programs of financial assistance to educational agencies, institutions and organizations; and for administering programs providing technical, consultative, and financial support to states, local communities, and other organizations and individuals in the provision of social, income maintenance, medical, and other services to the elderly and young.

DIAGNOSIS AND TREATMENT SERVICES—Diagnosis and treatment services are those intended to identify or alleviate specific diseases and conditions or their symptoms. Diagnostic and treatment services include:
- Obstetrical Services
- Surgical Services
- Diagnostic Radiology Services
- Therapeutic Radiology Services
- Clinical Laboratory Services
- Emergency Medical Services
- Dental Health Services
- Mental Health Services
- General Medical Services

EARLY AND PERIODIC SCREENING DIAGNOSIS AND TREATMENT PROGRAM (EPSDT)—A program mandated by law as part of the Medicaid program. It required that by July 1, 1969 all states have in effect a program for eligible children under 21 to ascertain their physical or mental condition and recommend required health care treatment.

EMERGENCY—A service component designed to provide 24 hour availability of psychiatric and other professional services for immediate intervention in personal crisis or other emergencies. The services are conducted under the direction of professional mental health personnel trained to assess the severity of the crisis and make use of appropriate community resources.

EMERGENCY MEDICAL SERVICE SYSTEM (EMSS)—An integrated system of appropriate health manpower, facilities and equipment intended to provide all necessary emergency care within a defined geographic area. This includes treatment on the site of accidents or other illness and transportation to appropriate health care facilities.

FEE-FOR-SERVICE—A free enterprise method used by physicians or other practitioners to charge for services as they are rendered. This is the usual method of billing by the majority of physicians in the United States. Under a fee-for-service payment system, expenditures increase not only if the fees increase but also if more units of service are delivered and charged for, or more expensive services are substituted for less expensive ones. This system contrasts with salary, per capita or prepayment systems and nationalized health care.

FINANCIAL FEASIBILITY—Technically defined as the ability of a health care provider to pay for the costs involved in capital investment and overall operation.

FULL DESIGNATION—A term applying to an organization that has been fully designated as a health systems agency by the Secretary of DHEW under P.L. 93-641. A health systems agency is fully designated when it has been empowered to perform all of the functions for which it was created.

GROUP PRACTICE—A formal association of three or more physicians or other health professionals providing services with income from medical practice pooled and redistributed in some prearranged fashion. Groups vary a great deal in size, composition, and financial arrangements.

HEALTH CARE SYSTEM—The network of professional health care services, consisting of professionals who provide services, facilities, and resources that support these services, financing mechanisms, the legal framework, and communications, and other relationships that link one part of the system to another.

HEALTH FACILITY—Usually a structure, including the physical plant and fixed equipment used in the provision of health services. Examples include hospitals, long-term organizations and ambulatory care centers.

HEALTH INSURANCE—Insurance against loss by disease or accidental bodily injury. Health insurance usually covers some of the medical costs of treating the disease or injury, may cover losses in earnings, and may be either an individual or group plan.

HEALTH MAINTENANCE ORGANIZATION (HMO)—An organized system of providing primary health care in a geographic area. An HMO accepts the responsibility to provide or assume the delivery of an agreed upon set of basic and supplemental health maintenance and treatment services to a voluntarily enrolled group of persons. For these services, the HMO is reimbursed through a predetermined, fixed, periodic prepayment. The HMO is responsible for providing most health and medical care services required by enrolled individuals or families. These services are specified in a contract between the HMO and those enrolled.

HEALTH MANPOWER—Collectively, all men and women working to provide health services to populations.

HEALTH RESOURCES—In health planning practice this term is generally defined as most of those resources used in producing health care services. They include capital, health manpower, health facilities, equipment, and supplies.

HEALTH SERVICE AREA—A geographic area deemed appropriate for the effective planning and development of health services. Legally, governors of the various states designate health service areas based on the following criteria: geography, political boundaries, population, health resources, and statewide coordination.

HEALTH SYSTEM—All the services, functions, resources, programs and financing mechanisms dealing with the health status of the population. The health planning legislation of 1974 requires health planning organizations to deal with the entire health care system in an organized, systematic fashion.

HEALTH SYSTEM ENABLING SERVICES—Organized activities designed to influence the means by which, and conditions under which, health systems services are delivered.

HEALTH SYSTEMS AGENCY (HSA)—A health planning and resources development agency designated under the terms of P.L. 93-641. HSA's functions include preparation of a health systems plan (HSP), an annual implementation plan (AIP), issuance of grants and contracts, the review and approval or disapproval of proposed uses of a wide range of federal funds in designated health service areas, and review of proposed new and existing institutional health services. Coordination is carried out on a statewide basis.

HEALTH SYSTEMS PLAN (HSP)—A document prepared annually by health systems agencies explaining the decisions reached by the organization pertaining to broad, strategic actions, and health resource changes recommended into approximately the next five years.

HOSPITAL—Institution whose primary function is to provide in-patient medical services. In addition, most hospitals provide some form of out-patient services, particularly emergency care. Hospitals are normally classified by length of stay (short-term or long-term); as teaching or nonteaching; by major type of service (psychiatric, tuberculosis, general, and other specialities); and by type of control (government, federal, state or local, not-for-profit, voluntary, etc.). The hospital system is dominated by the short-term, general, nonprofit community hospital, often called the voluntary hospital.

INPATIENT—A patient admitted for a minimum time of at least overnight to a hospital or other health care facility for the purpose of receiving diagnostic treatment or other health services.

INSTITUTIONAL HEALTH SERVICES—Health services delivered on an in-patient basis in hospitals, nursing homes, or other similar institutions, and by health maintenance organizations; however, recent definitions also include services delivered on an out-patient basis by departments or other organizational units of such institutions. The 1974 legislation defines these services as subject to DHEW rules according to Section 1122 review, including certificate of need requirements and assessments of appropriateness.

INTENSIVE CARE UNIT—A specialized unit in a hospital concentrating on seriously ill patients needing constant surveillance and nursing care. Some intensive care units limit services to either coronary care, intensive surgical care, and intensive care for newborn infants.

INTERMEDIATE CARE FACILITY—A nursing home or distinct part of a nursing home participating in Medicaid (Title XIX) as a general nursing care facility.

JOINT COMMISSION ON ACCREDITATION OF HOSPITALS (JCAH)—A private, nonprofit organization whose purpose is to encourage the attainment of uniformly high standards of institutional medical care. The JCAH, comprised of representatives of the American Hospital Association, the American Medical Association, the American College of Physicians, and the American College of Surgeons, establishes guidelines for the operation of hospitals and other health facilities and conducts surveys and accreditation programs.

LENGTH OF STAY—The length of stay for patients in hospitals and other health facilities. Length of stay is an important measure of the use of health facilities. It is usually reported as an average number of days spent in a facility per admission or discharge. It is calculated by taking the total number of days spent in a facility for all hospital discharges and deaths occurring during the time period divided by the number of discharges and deaths during the same period.

LONG–TERM CARE—Health and personal care services required by the chronically ill, aged, diabled, or sometimes retarded in an institution or at home on a long-term basis.

MEDICAID (TITLE XIX)—A federally aided, state operated and administered program providing medical coverage for specified low income persons. Authorized as part of the Social Security Act, Medicaid covers only the poor who are members of one of several categories of people included under welfare cash payment programs, the aged, the blind, the disabled, and members of families with dependent children where one parent is not present.

MEDICARE (TITLE XVIII)—A nationwide health insurance program for people 65 years of age and over, for persons eligible for Social Security disability payments for over two years, and for certain workers and their families who need specialized care such as kidney transplantation or dialysis.

NATIONAL HEALTH PLANNING AND RESOURCES DEVELOPMENT ACT OF 1974—This legislation consists of the addition of two new titles to the Public Health Service Act. Title XV establishes a new program for health planning and resources development, and Title XVI revises existing programs for the construction and modernization of health care facilities (the former Hill–Burton program) and authorizes funds for development of health resources.

OCCUPANCY RATE—A measure of in-patient health facility use determined by dividing available bed-days by patient-days. The occupancy rate is intended to measure the average percentage of a hospital's beds occupied.

OCCUPATIONAL HEALTH SERVICES—Health services concerned with the physical, mental, and social well-being of populations in relation to employment environment. In the United States, the principal federal statute concerned with occupational health is the Occupational Safety and Health Act administered by the Occupational Safety and Health Administration (OSHA) and the National Institute of Occupational Safety and Health (NIOSH).

OUTPATIENT—A patient receiving ambulatory care at a hospital or other health facility.

OUTPATIENT DEPARTMENT—An organized unit of a hospital with facilities and medical services exclusively or primarily devoted to those receiving ambulatory care.

PATIENT, INDIGENT—A patient whose income is poverty-level or below and eligible to receive some form of public assistance to pay all or part of his health care costs.

PATIENT, MEDICALLY INDIGENT—An individual who cannot affort the full cost of health care, but whose income is sufficient to make him ineligible for public assistance.

PATIENT ORIGIN STUDY—A geographical analysis used in determining the distributions of patients served by specific health care facilities or programs.

PREPAID GROUP PRACTICE—A formal association of three or more physicians providing a defined set of services over a specified period of time in return for a fixed, periodic prepayment made in advance.

PRIMARY CARE PHYSICIAN—General or family practice physicians, internists, pediatricians, obstetricians, and gynecologists.

PRIMARY HEALTH CARE—A broad array of preventive and rehabilitative services not primarily medical in nature. Included are such aspects as health education, nutrition, vocational rehabilitation, family planning, and social services.

PRIMARY MEDICAL CARE—Diagnostic and therapeutic care provided by physicians and registered nurses. It includes such services as immunization and physical examination and does not normally require the utilization of elaborate facilities or equipment generally associated with large medical centers or general hospitals.

PROVIDER—An individual or organization providing health care services in exchange for reimbursement from a purchaser.

RATE REVIEW—A system for the review of proposed charges (rates) of health care institutions to determine appropriateness. Proposed rate increases judged to be inappropriate by health planning agencies will not receive institutional reimbursement under insurance and similar payment mechanisms.

RESOURCES—The facilities, manpower, capital and knowledge required to accomplish a set of health care program objectives. Forecasts of resource requirements and ability have been incorporated into the current health care facilities planning programs.

SECTION 1122—This is a section of the Social Security Act providing that payment will not be made under Medicare or Medicaid if specified delivery mechanisms are inconsistent with state or local health plans. The 1974 health planning legislation requires that state health planning and development agencies serve as Section 1122 agencies for purposes of required reviews.

SHARED SERVICES—The coordinated or otherwise explicitly agreed upon sharing of responsibility for provision of health services by two or more otherwise independent hospitals or health care programs. The sharing of medical services might include, for example, an agreement that one hospital provide all pediatric care required in a community and another assume the responsibility for obstetrical care.

STATE HEALTH PLAN (SHP)—A statewide health plan intended to represent broad strategic actions and health resource changes recommended over a period extending a minimum of five years from the date of the plan. Included are recommendations for the implementation of the plan geared toward attaining explicitly stated goals and objectives.

STATE HEALTH PLANNING AND DEVELOPMENT AGENCY (SHPDA)—Section 1521 of P.L. 93-641 requires the establishment of state health planning and development agencies in each state. SHPDA's are tasked to prepare an annual preliminary state health plan and state medical facilities plan. The agency is also tasked to serve as the designated review agency for purposes of Section 1122 review and to administer a Certificate of Need Program.

STATE MEDICAL FACILITIES PLAN (SMFP)—A document presenting the decisions reached by the State Health Planning and Development Agency and approved by the Statewide Health Coordinating Council specifying state requirements for medical facilities, financial assistance for medical construction, modernization and conversion, and sets of priorities for such assistance.

STATEWIDE HEALTH COORDINATING COUNCIL (SHCC)—A state council of providers and consumers called for in the 1974 health planning legislation. Each SHCC is expected to generally supervise the work of state health planning and development agencies and review and coordinate plans and budgets of health systems agencies within states. It is also tasked to annually prepare a state health plan on the basis of local health systems agencies plans and preliminary plans of the state agency. The SHCC is also responsible for reviewing applications for HSA planning and resource development assistance.

THIRD PARTY PAYER—Any organization, public or private, that pays or insures health or medical expenses on behalf of beneficiaries or recipients (for example, Blue Cross and Blue Shield, commercial insurance companies, Medicare and Medicaid). Individuals generally pay a premium for such coverage in all private and some public programs. The organization then pays the bills in the form of third party payments.

UTILIZATION—Utilization is commonly defined in terms of patterns or rates of use of a health service facility. Measurement of utilization of medical services is normally accomplished in economic terms, but often expressed in rates per unit of population at risk for specified periods of time.

UTILIZATION REVIEW—Evaluation of the necessity, appropriateness, and efficiency of the use of medical services, procedures, and facilities. Hospital review includes appropriateness of admissions, lengths of stay, services offered, and discharge practice.

INDEX